Female Health Across the Lifespan

Editor

ALICE L. MARCH

NURSING CLINICS OF NORTH AMERICA

www.nursing.theclinics.com

Consulting Editor
STEPHEN D. KRAU

June 2018 • Volume 53 • Number 2

ELSEVIER

1600 John F. Kennedy Boulevard • Suite 1800 • Philadelphia, Pennsylvania, 19103-2899

http://www.theclinics.com

NURSING CLINICS OF NORTH AMERICA Volume 53, Number 2
June 2018 ISSN 0029-6465, ISBN-13: 978-0-323-58405-0

Editor: Kerry Holland
Developmental Editor: Casey Potter

Nursing Clinics of North America (ISSN 0029-6465) is published quarterly by Elsevier Inc., 360 Park Avenue South, New York, NY 10010-1710. Months of issue are March, June, September, and December. Periodicals postage paid at New York, NY and additional mailing offices. Subscription price per year is, $155.00 (US individuals), $465.00 (US institutions), $275.00 (international individuals), $567.00 (international institutions), $220.00 (Canadian individuals), $567.00 (Canadian institutions), $100.00 (US students), and $135.00 (international students). To receive student/resident rate, orders must be accompanied by name of affiliated institution, date of term, and the signature of program/residency coordinator on institution letterhead. Orders will be billed at individual rate until proof of status is received. Foreign air speed delivery is included in all *Clinics* subscription prices. All prices are subject to change without notice. **POSTMASTER:** Send address changes to *Nursing Clinics*, Elsevier Health Sciences Division, Subscription Customer Service, 3251 Riverport Lane, Maryland Heights, MO 63043. **Customer Service: Telephone:** 1-800-654-2452 (U.S. and Canada); **1-314-447-8871 (outside U.S. and Canada). Fax:** 1-314-447-8029. **E-mail: journalscustomerservice-usa@elsevier.com** (for print support) and **journalsonlinesupport-usa@elsevier.com** (for online support).

Nursing Clinics of North America is covered in *EMBASE/Excerpta Medica, MEDLINE/PubMed (Index Medicus), Social Sciences Citation Index, Current Contents, ASCA, Cumulative Index to Nursing, RNdex Top 100,* and Allied Health Literature and International Nursing Index (INI).

Contributors

CONSULTING EDITOR

STEPHEN D. KRAU, PhD, RN, CNE
Associate Professor (Retired), Vanderbilt University Medical Center, School of Nursing, Nashville, Tennessee, USA

EDITOR

ALICE L. MARCH, RN, PhD, FNP, CNE
Assistant Dean for Graduate Programs, Professor, Capstone College of Nursing, The University of Alabama, Tuscaloosa, Alabama, USA

AUTHORS

LEIGH BOOTH, EdD, RN
Assistant Professor, Capstone College of Nursing, The University of Alabama, Tuscaloosa, Alabama, USA

ELIZABETH KEELEY BOWMAN, RN, DNP, WHNP
Faculty/Assistant Professor, Vanderbilt University School of Nursing, Nashville, Tennessee, USA

ELIZABETH DI VALERIO, BS
Department of Biological Sciences, The University of Alabama, Tuscaloosa, Missouri, USA

SAFIYA GEORGE DALMIDA, PhD
Associate Professor, Assistant Dean for Research, Capstone College of Nursing, The University of Alabama, Tuscaloosa, Alabama, USA

KATHY GILL-HOPPLE, PhD, RN, SANE-A, SANE-P
Forensic Nurse Examiner Coordinator, Forensic Nursing Services, Medical University of South Carolina, Charleston, South Carolina, USA

ELIZABETH HALL, RN, APRN, DNP, WHNP-BC, SANE
Faculty/Instructor, Vanderbilt University School of Nursing, Nashville, Tennessee, USA

ASHLEY L. HODGES, PhD, CRNP, WHNP-BC
Associate Professor, Assistant Dean for Graduate Clinical Programs, Department of Family, Community, and Health Systems, University of Alabama at Birmingham School of Nursing, Birmingham, Alabama, USA

AIMEE CHISM HOLLAND, DNP, WHNP-BC, FNP-BC, RD
Associate Professor, DNP Program Director, Department of Family, Community, and Health Systems, University of Alabama at Birmingham School of Nursing, Birmingham, Alabama, USA

DEBRA HOLLOWAY, RGN, BA(Hons), MSc, FRCOG
Nurse Consultant, Gynaecology, Guy's and St Thomas' NHS Foundation Trust,
Mcnair Centre, Guy's Hospital, London, United Kingdom

NOLA HOLNESS, CNM, ARNP (Adult), MSN, PhD
Florida International University, Alexandria, Virginia, USA

MARCIA McDONNELL HOLSTAD, PhD
Emory University, Nell Hodgson Woodruff School of Nursing, Atlanta, Georgia, USA

GWENDOLYN L. HOOPER, PhD, FNP-BC, CUNP
Assistant Professor, Graduate Nursing, Capstone College of Nursing, The University of
Alabama, Tuscaloosa, Alabama, USA

HAROLD G. KOENIG, MD
Department of Psychiatry, Duke University Medical Center, Durham, North Carolina, USA;
Department of Medicine, King Abdulaziz University, Jeddah, Saudi Arabia

KYLE R. KRAEMER, MA
Department of Psychology, The University of Alabama, Tuscaloosa, Alabama, USA

ALICE L. MARCH, RN, PhD, FNP, CNE
Assistant Dean for Graduate Programs, Professor, Capstone College of Nursing,
The University of Alabama, Tuscaloosa, Alabama, USA

OLIVIA WINDHAM MAY, DNP, CRNP
Assistant Professor, Capstone College of Nursing, The University of Alabama,
Tuscaloosa, Alabama, USA

ANNE McKIBBIN, PhD, RN
Tuscaloosa County Domestic Violence Task Force, Tuscaloosa, Alabama, USA

JAYME MEJIA, RN, MS, FNP-C
Assistant Clinical Professor, Department of Family Health Care Nursing, University of
California, San Francisco, San Francisco, California, USA

ROBINGALE PANEPINTO, RN, DNP, FNP
Faculty/Instructor, Vanderbilt University School of Nursing, Nashville, Tennessee, USA

SUSAN JO ROBERTS, DNSc, ANP, FAAN
Professor, School of Nursing, Northeastern University, Boston, Massachusetts, USA

NAOMI A. SCHAPIRO, RN, PhD, CPNP-PC
Professor of Clinical Family Health Care Nursing, University of California, San Francisco,
San Francisco, California, USA

DIANE L. SPATZ, PhD, RN-BC, FAAN
Professor of Perinatal Nursing and the Helen M. Shearer Professor of Nutrition,
Department of Family and Community Health, University of Pennsylvania School
of Nursing, Nurse Researcher and Director of the Lactation Program, The Children's
Hospital of Philadelphia, Philadelphia, Pennsylvania, USA

ADELINE TURNER
Nursing Student, Capstone College of Nursing, The University of Alabama, Tuscaloosa,
Alabama, USA

STEPHEN UNGVARY, MA
Department of Psychology, The University of Alabama, Tuscaloosa, Alabama, USA

MONIKA WEDGEWORTH, EdD, RN, CNE
Assistant Professor, Capstone College of Nursing, The University of Alabama, Tuscaloosa, Alabama, USA

Contents

Section I: Childhood

> Urinary tract infection is one of the most common bacterial infections in infants and young children. There are 5 collection methods commonly used to obtain a urine sample from an infant or small child: suprapubic aspiration, urethral catheterization, clean catch void, urine collection bag, and urine collection pad. Although suprapubic aspiration and urethral catheterization are invasive, they are less likely to cause contamination of the specimen. When deciding which method to use, providers must take into consideration the clinical presentation of a child, as well as presenting and past medical history, while weighing benefits versus risks.

Section II: Adolescence

> Adolescent access to reproductive health services, mental health services, and treatment of drug and alcohol use depends on teens' rights to consent and confidentiality in the state in which they live. This article reviews the history, current practices, and potential challenges to confidentiality, including Title X funding, questions about brain development and ability to make autonomous choices, and meaningful use practices in electronic records. Resources are provided for professional position statements and individual state regulations.

> According to the World Health Organization, 10% to 13% of postpartum women develop a mental disorder, mainly depression. This number is higher in developing countries. This percentage increases in adolescents, and symptoms in adolescents tend to be overlooked. These disorders can be treated successfully if detected early, which will in turn prevent more severe symptoms from developing. This article provides evidence-based clinical best practices for the assessment and early recognition of postpartum depression, specifically in adolescents. In addition, suggestions for integration into practice and recommendations for interprofessional collaboration are discussed.

Section III: Common to Childbearing-Aged Women

Preconception counseling is essential for women of childbearing age and family members who have decided to conceive because the level of well health of the mother and unborn child are affected by decisions and actions of the mother before and during pregnancy. Proactively planning pregnancy includes scheduling a preconception counseling consultation with a provider. Understanding physical, psychological, and emotional needs promotes healthy pregnancy outcomes for mother and baby. This article offers a reflective and holistic perspective of how health care providers frame, prioritize, and engage with the patient and family during the preconception consultation.

Intimate partner violence (IPV) is a health epidemic. Health care professionals have a unique and critical role to play. It is expected that health care providers have the ability to engage in an informed response to IPV, which is crucial to the safety of the woman, improving health outcomes and preventing further violence. Screening procedures for IPV, along with the awareness of abuse indicators, have the potential to significantly identify women who have been exposed to IPV. Identification of IPV will enable the health care provider to offer support, build trust, validate concerns, and offer community resources.

The spread of sexually transmitted infections (STIs) remains a significant public health issue in the United States. Social, economic, and behavioral implications affecting the spread of STIs have been identified. The most important social factor in the United States is the stigma associated with discussing sex and STI screening. In this article, specific recommendations for women are included regarding screening, diagnosing, and treating common vaginal and cervical infections. Screening women for infections of the vagina and cervix is essential because untreated infections may result in complications that have current and long-term health consequences and affect quality of life.

This study examined factors affecting the psychological well-being of women living with human immunodeficiency virus/AIDS and the impact of depression on clinical outcomes. Nearly two-thirds of participants in this cross-sectional study reported significant depressive symptoms. Compared with women living with human immunodeficiency virus/AIDS without depressive symptoms, those with depression reported significantly poorer health outcomes. Health care providers should regularly screen these women for and adequately treat depression and must collaborate with mental health providers and pastoral care counselors to address the mental health needs of women living with human immunodeficiency virus/AIDS to optimize their human immunodeficiency virus–related outcomes.

Health Care of Sexual Minority Women

Susan Jo Roberts

Sexual minority women may be invisible in health care settings unless practitioners ask every patient about sexual attractions/behaviors and identity. Sexual minority women need to feel comfortable and be able to share information about their sexual identity, partners, and lives. No medical diagnoses are found more commonly in sexual minority women, but problems such as overweight/obesity, increased tobacco and alcohol use, increased mental health problems, and a past history of childhood sexual abuse are common. These factors intertwine when treating sexual minority women.

High-Risk Pregnancy

Nola Holness

Any unexpected or unanticipated medical or obstetric condition associated with a pregnancy with an actual or potential hazard to the health or well-being of the mother or fetus is considered a high-risk pregnancy. There is no exact definition of risk in pregnancy, as risk may be perceived in different ways by the woman and her health care provider. Women with complicated pregnancies may require lifestyle changes, medication regimens, technical support, and even hospitalization. Nurses can foster an environment of security and trust during preconception, antenatal, intrapartal, and postnatal care to enhance the health and well-being of the mother and fetus.

Helping Mothers Reach Personal Breastfeeding Goals

Diane L. Spatz

Professional organizations worldwide recommend exclusive human milk/breastfeeding for the first 6 months of life, and continued breastfeeding with appropriate complementary foods for 1 year or more. This article focuses on the importance of prenatal messaging and goal setting to ensure that mothers are able to optimize their milk supply during the critical window of opportunity in first 2 weeks after delivery. Research data in the United States indicate that the largest categories of why women stopped breastfeeding were for reasons related to milk supply or concerns that the infant was not getting enough nutrition or gaining enough weight.

Section IV: Older Adult

Menopause Symptom Management in the United Kingdom

Debra Holloway

Menopause is a complex time in a woman's life. It is increasingly a midlife event, when health care professionals should be aiming to optimize a woman's health for the next 30 years or so. Nurses need to be able to give up-to-date information and evidence for all forms of treatment based on a background of complex and ever-changing research. This article covers the main presenting complaints and treatments, from lifestyle to hormone replacement therapy, by drawing on guidelines from national bodies.

In the United States, people older than 65 years attend approximately 248 million health care visits each year, or 7 visits per older adult annually. One in every 5 older adults reports recent sexual activity, yet health care professionals do not ask, and patients do not tell, when it comes to sexuality. The desire to engage in sex and intimate behaviors to meet important quality-of-life needs is present in people of all ages. Because it is important to communicate in a nonjudgmental manner, health care professionals must first examine their own personal attitudes and values regarding sexuality in older women.

Pelvic organ prolapse is a common condition affecting women of any age but more likely to occur in the aging woman. Prolapse has a significant impact on quality of life, sexuality, and body image. Vaginal support pessaries have been used since ancient times and are a safe and effective nonsurgical treatment option. Fitting a pessary results in immediate symptom improvement. A comprehensive evaluation for pessary fitting is time intensive but necessary. Nurse providers perform direct pessary care and have a role in caring for women with prolapse expanding access to care. Caregiver and family involvement is important for pessary care and follow-up.

NURSING CLINICS OF NORTH AMERICA

THE CLINICS ARE AVAILABLE ONLINE!
Access your subscription at:
www.theclinics.com

Preface

Female Health Across the Lifespan

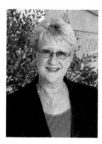

Alice L. March, RN, PhD, FNP, CNE
Editor

In the United States, more women than men seek health care each year. In 2015, 89.2% of women reported a visit to a health care professional within the past 12 months, as opposed to 77.8% of men.[1] Before the age of 65 years, women also spend more on health care annually than men ($4673 vs $3835, respectively). Yet, after age 65, the numbers are reversed (women = $9859 vs men = $10,471).[2] Even though women in the United States are seen more often and spend more health care dollars, the health-spending efficiency by gender in the United States ranks 25th out of 27 high-income countries in reducing women's death rates.[3] To answer the question of why this gender inequality may exist, it is important to examine the history of how the United States to came to provide women's health care across the lifespan.

Michelle Obama (Ted Conferences, 2009) said, "Communities and countries and ultimately the world are only as strong as the health of their women." This quote reinforces the values, beliefs, and norms related to the health and health care of women that have changed dramatically since the beginning of the twentieth century. In 1916, even though few women worked outside of the home, one of Theodore Roosevelt's campaign promises was a health insurance plan that would provide maternity benefits for women workers.[4] Later in the century, during the 1960s and 1970s, feminists made a clear connection between the health care system and the treatment of women by highlighting the epidemic of unnecessary hysterectomies, while other women (without access to primary care) died of preventable cervical and uterine cancers. In 1973, the need for safe abortions and privacy was brought before the Supreme Court, and women were afforded the right to privacy in reproductive health care and to legal abortion services. During the 1990s, a strong push for health reform was mounted. This was specifically directed at the inclusion of primary and preventive services, particularly full reproductive health care and family planning.[4] Finally, in the twenty-first century, the passage of the Affordable Care Act instituted preventative care benefits for women, to be provided without copay or coinsurance. This includes

Nurs Clin N Am 53 (2018) xiii–xiv
https://doi.org/10.1016/j.cnur.2018.03.001
0029-6465/18/© 2018 Published by Elsevier Inc.

various services throughout the lifespan of women from pregnancy testing and breast-feeding support to mammograms and osteoporosis screening.[5]

Nurses, as formal and informal educators, must be prepared to provide basic information, as well as specialized knowledge to patients and to nursing students. This collection of articles spans the lifecycle of women, from childhood urinary tract infections to care of sexual minority women, and sexuality in the older adult woman. In this issue, you will find current information from practicing nurses, advanced practitioners, and active nurse educators about young women as teenage mothers and the often underdiagnosed issue of postpartum depression as well as consent and privacy issues in adolescents. The selections related to women of childbearing age include intimate partner violence screening information, sexually transmitted infection diagnosis and treatment, and information about the effect of depression on medication adherence and quality of life among women living with HIV and AIDS. Specific to pregnancy, there are review articles about preconception planning, high-risk pregnancy, and lactation. The collection concludes with some considerations relevant to the older adult woman: menopause symptom management, pessary fitting and care, and sexuality among older adult women.

The authors and I hope this concise collection will aid you in the care of the women you will encounter as you teach students, and as you care for patients of all ages.

Alice L. March, RN, PhD, FNP, CNE
The University of Alabama
Capstone College of Nursing
Box 870358
Tuscaloosa, AL 35487, USA

E-mail address:
almarch@ua.edu

REFERENCES

1. National Health Interview Survey. Blackwell DL, Villaroel MA. Tables of summary health statistics for US adults: 2015 National Health Interview Survey. National Center for Health Statistics. 2016. Available at: http://www.cdc.gov/nchs/nhis/SHS/tables.htm. Accessed November 30, 2017. NCHS, National Health Interview Survey; 2015.
2. National Center for Health Statistics. Health, United States, 2016; with chartbook on long-term trends in health. Hyattsville (MD): Centers for Disease Control and Prevention; 2017.
3. US Ranks near bottom among industrialized nations in efficiency of health care spending. UCLA Fielding School of Public Health, 12 December 2013. Available at: https://ph.ucla.edu/news/press-release/2013/dec/us-ranks-near-bottom-among-industrialized-nations-efficiency-health-care. Accessed November 30, 2017.
4. Hoffman B. Health care reform and social movements in the United States. Am J Public Health 2003;92(1):75–85.
5. Preventative care benefits for women. Available at: https://www.healthcare.gov/preventive-care-women/. Accessed November 30, 2017.

Section I: Childhood

Urine Collection Methods in Children: Which is the Best?

Olivia Windham May, DNP, CRNP

KEYWORDS

- Urine collection • Urinalysis • Pediatrics • Children • Urinary tract infection

KEY POINTS

- Urinary tract infection is one of the most common bacterial infections in infants and young children.
- There are 5 commonly used methods to obtain a urine specimen from an infant or young child: suprapubic aspiration, urethral catheterization, clean catch void, urine collection bag, and urine collection pad.
- Suprapubic aspiration and urethral catheterization are invasive but more reliable than the other methods when obtaining an accurate urine sample.
- Urinalysis and urine culture may not substitute for each other in the diagnosis of urinary tract infection in the pediatric population.

Urinary tract infection (UTI) is one of the most common bacterial infections in infants and young children, especially girls. Accurate and early diagnosis is essential to avoid long-term complications, such as hydronephrosis or permanent renal scarring, from under-treatment or delayed treatment of pyelonephritis and unnecessary treatments, such as antibiotics, invasive procedures, and radiographic studies. The diagnosing of UTI can be difficult when based on history and physical examination alone, because most young, nonverbal children present with fever as the only symptom and assessment finding. In addition to fever, older children may come to a clinic with vomiting, loose stools, and abdominal or flank pain. Cystitis and pyelonephritis are more likely in older children.[1]

Infants and young children are more likely to have bacteremia and/or sepsis than older children, and accurate diagnosis and appropriate treatment are essential for this age group. Febrile infant girls are twice as likely to have a UTI as febrile infant boys. Uncircumcised boys are 4 time to 20 times more likely to have a UTI than circumcised boys.[2] The likelihood of a UTI is significantly reduced when another

There are no funding sources, commercial or financial conflicts of interest for the author of this article.
Capstone College of Nursing, The University of Alabama, PO Box 870358, Tuscaloosa, AL 35487, USA
E-mail address: omay@ua.edu

clinically obvious source of infection is observed, placing further importance on the role of the urinalysis in the diagnosis. There are 5 common methods to obtain urine specimens from children for urinalysis and culture. Invasive techniques include suprapubic aspiration (SPA) and urethral catheterization, and noninvasive techniques include urine bags, collection pads, and clean catch void.[3] There are advantages and disadvantages to each method.

ROLE OF THE URINALYSIS AND URINE CULTURE

Diagnostic testing for a UTI begins with the simple urinalysis and urine culture. Clinical practice guidelines from the American Academy of Pediatrics (AAP)[2] recommend the following for children ages 2 months to 24 months (**Box 1**). A simple urine dipstick provides rapid results, which makes it useful in the presumptive diagnosis of a UTI. Nitrites are produced by the bacterial conversion of nitrates, which are present in the normal flora of urine. Most UTI-causing gram-negative bacteria are capable of producing nitrites, but not all UTIs are caused by gram-negative bacteria. Children who empty their bladders frequently, especially infants, may have a false-negative result. Therefore, the test for nitrites has a low sensitivity but high specificity for the diagnosis of UTI in the pediatric population.[4] Nitrite presence is suggestive of UTI but its absence does not rule out a diagnosis.

The leukocyte esterase test has a 94% sensitivity when used for a suspected UTI. Although it is rare, it is possible for a child to have a UTI without the presence of pyuria. White blood cells can be found in the urine with Kawasaki disease, streptococcal infections, and vigorous exercise. Therefore, pyuria cannot confirm that an infection is present. A microscopic examination of the urine and a culture should follow even when the simple urinalysis is negative for leukocytes.[2] Asymptomatic bacteriuria occurs when low virulent bacteria colonize the urinary tract without causing inflammation. This is common in infant and school-aged girls. The presence of pyuria can help distinguish asymptomatic bacteriuria from a true UTI. Antibiotic therapy for asymptomatic bacteriuria is not necessary.

A urine culture is the most definitive way to diagnose a UTI, and the final result, positive or negative, can be affected by the method of collection. The perineal area and distal urethra are normally colonized with fecal bacteria, which make contamination of the specimen likely when obtained by a collection pad or bag.[4] A negative result can confirm that a UTI is not present when obtained using one of these methods. There is also the possibility that a culture may produce a low colony count when the specimen is collected through a clean catch void (CCV) or catheterization, even

---

Box 1
Criteria for diagnosing a urinary tract infection in infants and children ages 2 months to 24 months

1. Positive urinalysis: dipstick testing positive for leukocyte esterase and/or nitrites, or microscopic examination detects white blood cells or bacteria

2. Positive urine culture: at least 50,000 colony-forming units per milliliter (1 species)

3. Both an abnormal urinalysis and a positive culture are needed to confirm inflammation/infection

Data from American Academy of Pediatrics. Urinary tract infection: Clinical practice guideline for the diagnosis and management of the initial UTI in febrile infants and children 2 to 24 months. Pediatrics 2011;128(3):595–610.

though bacteria is not present in the urine itself. To declare a urine culture positive, there must be a minimum of 50,000 colony-forming units per milliliter of a single urinary pathogen.[2] Obtaining a urine specimen from an infant or young child can be difficult, further increasing the possibility of contamination during the procedure. Because of this, health care providers must weigh the benefits and risks of each collection method in addition to obtaining a very thorough history and physical.

METHODS FOR COLLECTION
Suprapubic Aspiration

SPA is considered the gold standard for urine collection to diagnose a UTI, especially in the non–toilet-trained population. SPA is a sterile procedure, which involves the use of a needle to aspirate urine directly from the bladder. This method reduces the possibility of contamination from the skin or distal urethra, which is common with other urine collection techniques. SPA can be performed with or without ultrasound guidance, although the use of ultrasound increases the success rate.[5] The indications for SPA are listed in **Box 2**.

SPA is contraindicated if a child is not fully hydrated, has an empty or nonpalpable bladder, has urinated within 1 hour prior to the procedure, has a suspected or actual intestinal obstruction, or has abdominal scars or wounds.[6] SPA is a specialized procedure and is not within the scope of practice of most registered nurses, even though they are the most likely professional to be charged with the task of obtaining the urine specimen. Although SPA is recommended in official practice guidelines, the actual collection of urine via SPA is rare. The procedure is considered invasive and painful, which can be a deterrent for health care providers and parents.[7]

Urethral Catheterization

Catheterization of the bladder is more commonly used when a sterile urine specimen is needed to diagnose a UTI. Although the procedure is invasive and can cause discomfort, it is more readily acceptable over an SPA and can easily be performed by a nurse in a hospital or outpatient clinic. Urine obtained through catheterization has a culture sensitivity of 95% and a specificity of 99%, making it an acceptable alternative when an SPA is not possible.[2] When obtaining urine through catheterization, clinicians should discard the first few drops of urine to lessen the likelihood of contamination from bacteria in the distal urethra. This is not always possible, however, because many urethral catheters are manufactured as part of a closed system.

Box 2
Indications for suprapubic aspiration collection

1. Sterile urine specimen needed

2. Frequent diarrheal stools

3. Male child with moderate or severe phimosis

4. Female child with tight labial adhesions

5. Urinary retention

Data from American Academy of Pediatrics. Urinary tract infection: Clinical practice guideline for the diagnosis and management of the initial UTI in febrile infants and children 2 to 24 months. Pediatrics 2011;128(3):595–610; and Plaza-Verduin MA, Lucas J. Suprapubic bladder aspiration. In: Ganti L, editor. Atlas of emergency medicine procedures. New York: Springer Verlag; 2016. p. 717–20.

A closed system lessens the possibility of contamination through transfer of a specimen or breaking of sterile technique.

Although catheterization is considered less invasive, it still can cause discomfort to a child. A child who is noncooperative can make the procedure more emotionally and physically traumatic. To decrease discomfort, clinicians should consider the option of applying 2% lidocaine jelly to the perimeatal area in female children. It takes approximately 3 minutes for the anesthetic to take effect.[8] Visualizing landmarks for the procedure can be difficult when performed on a young girl, making catheterization of the vagina a common event. If this occurs, the catheter should be left in place to serve as a landmark and a second catheter inserted into the urethral meatus. Clinicians often fail to do this, increasing the possibility of contamination of the specimen from bacteria in the vagina. Contraindications to urethral catheterization are shown in **Box 3**.

Clean Catch Void

The CCV method has distinct advantages over more invasive methods for obtaining a urine specimen. A CCV can be used in a variety of inpatient and outpatient settings and does not rely on the technical skills of a clinician. Obtaining a true midstream specimen from a young child can be difficult. The main negative consideration associated with a CCV is higher rates of contamination from fecal matter and bacteria on the skin of the perineal area (16%–38%).[9] This sometimes leads to unnecessary antibiotic treatment, radiological studies, or repeated urine testing using more invasive techniques. Although the basics of the procedure are consistent across settings, there is significant variability in the actual practice of the techniques used. The role of the collector, cleaning solutions, and methods differ by facility and setting. Parents frequently are asked to collect a specimen and may find the procedure messy and time-consuming. In addition, parents are more likely to touch the container against the perineal skin, contaminate the inside of the sterile container, or not catch the specimen midstream for fear of getting urine on their hands.[10] The value of this collection method is primarily to rule out a UTI rather than diagnose one.

Urine Collection Bag

The sterile urine collection bag is a common method used to obtain a urine specimen from a non–toilet-trained child, namely infants and younger toddlers. Because

---

Box 3
Contraindications to urethral catheterization in infants and children

1. Female child with tight labial adhesions

2. Child with a pelvic injury

3. Known trauma to the urethra

4. Male child with moderate or severe phimosis

5. Child with visible blood at the urethral meatus

Data from American Academy of Pediatrics. Urinary tract infection: clinical practice guideline for the diagnosis and management of the initial UTI in febrile infants and children 2 to 24 months. Pediatrics 2011;128(3):595–610; and Plaza-Verduin MA, Lucas J. Suprapubic bladder aspiration. In: Ganti L, editor. Atlas of emergency medicine procedures. New York: Springer Verlag; 2016. p. 717–20.

the method is noninvasive, many health care providers prefer it over urethral catheterization and SPA, regardless of the potential for contamination. A sterile urine collection bag is applied to the perineum after cleansing the skin. Cleaning solutions vary between facilities but the procedure is consistent. There is significant risk of contamination from bacteria on the skin of the perineal area, and fecal matter may inadvertently enter the collection bag. When a collection bag fills with urine, it becomes heavy and typically pulls away from the skin. Besides loss of specimen, this allows bacteria to enter from the diaper itself if worn at the same time. A positive culture from a specimen obtained through a collection bag is false positive 88% of the time.[2]

Urine Collection Pad

The urine collection pad is a noninvasive, cost-efficient, and easy method for obtaining a urine specimen from non–toilet-trained infants and children. A parent or clinician must clean the diaper area with chlorhexidine or another cleaning substance and then apply a clean diaper with the pad inserted. Once the child voids, a sterile syringe is used to aspirate a minimum of 0.5 mL of urine from the pad. The pad must not be visibly soiled from feces because this has the potential for contamination.[3] Benefits of the urine collection pad include timely specimen collection, less trauma to the child, and increased parental satisfaction. The method does have, however, a high rate of contamination, similar to the CCV and urine collection bag methods. Contamination can occur from feces and from organisms on the skin. Children with diaper rashes should not have urine collected in this manner.

WHAT THE GUIDELINES SAY

In 2011, the AAP released updated guidelines for the diagnosis and management of UTIs in children 2 months to 24 months of age.[2] Data from recent publications were graded and analysis of the literature occurred to outline current evidence-based research. Regarding urine collection methods, for ill-appearing febrile infants with no apparent source of infection, the AAP recommends that urine be obtained through urethral catheterization or SPA.[2] Review of the literature does not support the use of a collection bag for this age group because of the high potential for contamination.[2] If it is determined by a clinician that a child is nontoxic in appearance, urine may be collected in the most convenient means available (CCV, urine collection bag, and so forth). In this scenario, if urinalysis results suggest a UTI, urine can be recollected by means of catheterization or SPA and then cultured. If urinalysis of fresh urine (<1 hour since void/collection) is negative for leukocyte esterase and nitrites, the clinician may withhold antimicrobial therapy and monitor the child for worsening condition.[2]

A urinalysis suggestive of infection and a positive urine culture are necessary to diagnose a true UTI. Therefore, one cannot be substituted for the other. The urinalysis may be predictive or presumptive of UTI but a diagnosis cannot be confirmed until the urine culture results are available. When initiating antimicrobial therapy, clinicians should take into consideration a child's past history and patterns of sensitivity for the local area and should then adjust therapy based on final culture sensitivity results. Antimicrobials should be prescribed for no less than 7 days. For ill-appearing or toxic patients who are unable to tolerate oral medications, 24 hours to 48 hours of parenteral therapy may be warranted (**Table 1**). Cephalosporins, amoxicillin plus clavulanic acid, and trimethoprim/sulfamethoxazole remain the usual empiric antimicrobial choices.

Table 1
Empiric antibiotics for the management of childhood urinary tract infection

Antibiotic	Dosage
Amoxicillin/clavulanate	20–45 mg/kg/d po divided q12h; 20–40 mg/kg/d po divided q8h
Ceftriaxone	50–100 mg/kg IM/IV divided q12–24h; max 4 g/24 h
Cefotaxime	Infants/children <50 kg: 75–200 mg/kg/d IM/IV divided q6–8h; max 12 g/d
Cefixime	6 mo–12 y, <45 kg: 8 mg/kg/d po divided qd–bid 6 mo–adult, >45 kg: 400 mg po qd; 200 mg po bid
Cefpodoxime	2 mo–11 y: 10 mg/kg/d po divided q12h × 5–10 d 12 y and older: 100–400 mg po bid × 7–14 d; max 800 mg/d
Cephalexin	25–50 mg/kg/d po divided q6–12h; max 4000 mg/24 h May give 50–100 mg/kg/d po divided q6h for severe infection >15 y old: 500 mg po q12h × 7–14 d
Gentamicin	8 d–23 mo: 2.5 mg/kg IV/IM q8h[a] 2 y and older: 2–2.5 mg/kg IV/IM q8h[a]
Trimethoprim/ sulfamethoxazole	2–23 mo: 8–12 mg/kg/d TMP po divided q6–12h × 7–14 d; max 320 mg/d TMP 2 y and older (mild–moderate infection): 8 mg/kg/d TMP po/IV divided q12h × 3–10 d

[a] Adjust dose based on levels.
Note: Dosage information obtained from ePocrates mobile application.[11]
Abbreviations: IM, intramuscular; IV, intravenous; max, maximum; TMP, trimethoprim.

SUMMARY

Clinical practice guidelines are clear when recommending urine collection methods for infants and young children. The decision by clinicians to follow those guidelines becomes cloudier when it comes to invasive procedures. In theory, obtaining a urine sample by SPA from an infant is a simple procedure with much accuracy. Yet it is an invasive procedure, which can be traumatic for infants and parents. The same applies to urethral catheterization, although less discomfort is expected and a 2% lidocaine jelly can be applied prior to the procedure. Parents are often likely to refuse a procedure when it has the potential to cause discomfort or pain. When deciding which method to use, a health care provider must take into consideration the clinical presentation of the child as well as present and past medical histories. Benefits of the procedure must outweigh the risks and those must be communicated to parents in a clear and convincing way.

REFERENCES

1. Habib S. Highlights for management of a child with a urinary tract infection. Int J Pediatr 2012;2012:1–6.
2. American Academy of Pediatrics. Urinary tract infection: clinical practice guideline for the diagnosis and management of the initial UTI in febrile infants and children 2 to 24 months. Pediatrics 2011;128(3):595–610.
3. Ho I, Lee CH, Fry M. A prospective comparative pilot study comparing the urine collection pad with clean catch urine technique in non-toilet-trained children. Int Emerg Nurs 2013;22(2):94–7.
4. Tsai JD, Lin CC, Yang SS. Diagnosis of pediatric urinary tract infections. Urol Sci 2016;3:131–4.

5. Ponka D, Baddar F. Suprapubic bladder aspiration. Can Fam Physician 2013; 59(1):50. Available at: http://www.cfpc.ca/CanadianFamilyPhysician/.

6. Plaza-Verduin MA, Lucas J. Suprapubic bladder aspiration. In: Ganti L, editor. Atlas of emergency medicine procedures. New York: Springer Verlag; 2016. p. 717–20. https://doi.org/10.1007/978-1-4939-2507-0.

7. Eliacik K, Kanik A, Yavascan O, et al. A comparison of bladder catheterization and suprapubic aspiration methods for urine sample collection from infants with a suspected urinary tract infection. Clin Pediatr 2016;55(9):819–24.

8. Robson W, Leung A, Thomason M. Catheterization of the bladder in infants and children. Clin Pediatr 2006;9:795–800.

9. Teo S, Cheek JA, Craig S. Improving clean-catch contamination rates: a prospective interventional cohort study. Emerg Med Australas 2016;28(6):698–703.

10. Karacan C, Erkek N, Senel S, et al. Evaluation of urine collection methods for the diagnosis of urinary tract infections in children. Med Princ Pract 2009;19(3): 188–91.

11. Epocrates Plus. Epocrates medical reference (Version 17.10) [Mobile application software]. 2017. Available at: http://itunes.apple.com. Accessed September 20, 2017.

Section II: Adolescence

Adolescent Confidentiality and Women's Health

History, Rationale, and Current Threats

Naomi A. Schapiro, RN, PhD, CPNP-PC*, Jayme Mejia, RN, MS, FNP-C

KEYWORDS

- Adolescent • Adolescent development • Adolescent health services
- Confidentiality/legislation and jurisprudence • Health services accessibility
- Patient rights/legislation and jurisprudence

KEY POINTS

- Consent and confidentiality are core components of adolescent health care.
- Legal and ethical precedents support autonomous adolescent decision making.
- Nurses must understand complex confidentiality and mandatory reporting regulations in their settings.
- Electronic health records and billing systems can improve or compromise confidentiality, and nurses should be aware of their own systems' capabilities and safeguards.
- Title X funding may be the only source of confidential reproductive care in some states.

An adolescent woman's access to confidentiality or privacy in reproductive care and her ability to consent to or make autonomous decisions about reproductive care and related emotional issues are core issues in her overall access to preventive care. This article reviews current statistics related to sexual activity and other adolescent risk issues and reviews the legal and ethical background to adolescent consent and confidentiality. Recent advances in neuroscience, electronic health records (EHRs), and funding streams for reproductive care that improve or impede confidential access to care are reviewed, with recommendations for nurses working with adolescents.

PROFESSIONAL ORGANIZATIONS AND CONFIDENTIALITY

The World Health Organization,[1] the United Nations Children's Fund,[2] the American Academy of Pediatrics,[3] the Association of Women's Health, Obstetric and Neonatal

---

Dr N.A. Schapiro has no financial interests to disclose. Ms J. Mejia is a Nexplanon trainer for Merck.
Department of Family Health Care Nursing, University of California San Francisco, 2 Koret Way, Rm N-411Y, San Francisco, CA 94143-0606, USA
* Corresponding author.
E-mail address: naomi.schapiro@ucsf.edu

Nurses,[4] and the Society for Adolescent Health and Medicine[5] all have policies supporting adolescent confidential access to reproductive health services (**Table 1**). In addition, *Bright Futures,*[6] published by the American Academy of Pediatrics, with partial support from the US Department of Health and Human Services and input from nursing, sets guidelines for pediatric and adolescent services. The 4th and current edition of *Bright Futures* recommends that pediatric practices develop formal confidentiality policies, which are explained to parents and to children by ages 7 to 8, and, that starting before or at the 12-year-old well-child visit, early adolescents should have dedicated time with their pediatric provider, without a parent in the room. *Bright Futures* also recommends discussions about sexual attraction, advantages of delaying sexual activity, contraception, sexually transmitted infection (STI) prevention and screening, and specific care for youth who are lesbian, gay, bisexual, transgender, questioning, or gender nonconforming.[6]

LEGAL AND ETHICAL ISSUES UNDERPINNING ADOLESCENT CONFIDENTIALITY

Until the twentieth century, children in the United States were considered "chattels" of their parents, without independent rights.[7] The concept of a mature minor, able to understand and consent to some medical procedures, evolved in the 1970s and 1980s. In 1967, the Supreme Court recognized that the due process clause of the 14th Amendment to the Constitution applied to children as well,[8] and by the late 1970s, several Supreme Court rulings acknowledged a right to privacy for adolescent consent to contraception and abortion.[7] Court rulings generally do not specify the determinants of whether a particular minor is mature enough to consent, although subsequent laws may specify a minimum age.[7,9] Twenty-six states allow minors to consent to general medical care if they are living apart from parents, either because of explicit law or because the state allows minors to consent to some or all medical care.[9,10] Minors may be considered to have many rights of adulthood, or emancipation, depending on the state, if they are married, if they are serving in the military, if they have gone to court seek emancipation, or in some states by declaration of parents.[9] In general, the mature and emancipated minor laws are exceptions, because US legal policy recognizes that human rights belong to adults rather than children, and this legal tradition may explain some of the resistance to the international Convention on the Rights of the Child,[2] which the United States has never ratified[10] (see **Table 1**).

Nursing articles about adolescent confidential services[11–13] have stressed principles of biomedical ethics,[14] such as autonomy, nonmaleficence, beneficence, and

Table 1	
Adolescent confidentiality policies	
Organization	**Year of Publication**
Association of Women's Health, Obstetric and Neonatal Nurses http://www.jognn.org/article/S0884-2175(15)30258-6/pdf	2010
American Academy of Pediatrics http://pediatrics.aappublications.org/content/138/2/e20161347.long	2016
Society for Adolescent Health and Medicine http://www.jahonline.org/article/S1054-139X%2804%2900086-2/fulltext	2004
World Health Organization http://apps.who.int/iris/bitstream/10665/102539/1/9789241506748_eng.pdf	2014
United Nations Children's Fund Convention on the Rights of the Child http://www.ohchr.org/EN/ProfessionalInterest/Pages/CRC.aspx	1989

justice, as well as legal precedents for confidentiality.[11,13] International policies, such as the Convention on the Rights of the Child[2] and the World Health Organization's policy on access to contraception,[1] stress the individual human rights of children and adolescents. US professional organizations have endorsed access to confidentiality and support the ability of adolescents to exercise autonomous decision making (see **Table 1**). With increasing research about adolescent neurologic, cognitive, and emotional development and their interactions,[15] however, the concept of the mature minor in specific and the adolescent's ability to make autonomous decisions in general have come into question.

According to Beauchamp and Childress,[14] autonomy, or self-rule, depends on freedom from external or internal controls, the capacity of an individual to understand the choice in question, and the implications of the various options. Although these philosophers do not endorse any particular test of competency or specify the age at which children become autonomous in decision making, their criteria are similar to those of the MacArthur competency tests (discussed later). These ethicists also stress a real-life, rather than ideal, definition, noting that individuals are rarely completely free of internal or external pressures when making decisions. They do not specifically discuss adolescent confidentiality, but they view the right to privacy, which has been the chief underpinning in US law for the right to make decisions about contraception,[16] as closely related to autonomous decision making.[14]

Children's competence to understand the implications and details of medical treatment have been evaluated more closely for research than clinical practice.[17] The MacArthur Competence Assessment Tool for Clinical Research (MacCAT-CR)[18] and the MacCAT-T,[19] developed for adults, test 4 domains of decision-making competence: comprehension of information about research, reasoning ability to decide on participation with an understanding of the available alternatives, appreciation of the effects of a particular treatment, and ability to express a choice about participating. In a study of children who were eligible for clinical research, the MacCAT-CR, a semistructured questionnaire, was found an adequate measure of the 4 domains.[20] In general, children 11.2 years and older were judged competent to make decisions, whereas children 9.6 years or younger were not judged competent, with varying results between those ages.[20] Other researchers have shown that scores on the MacCAT-CR are higher in adolescents from more affluent backgrounds and higher degrees of health literacy.[21]

In recent literature about adolescent decision-making ability, there have been 2 schools of thought.[22] The 2 factions include those who promote the autonomy of the child by advocating for lower age of consent and those who advocate for a more conservative approach to consent to protect the child. Although cognitive processes and cognitive tests, such as the MacArthur tests, discussed previously, indicate that children have the capacity to make research and some medical decisions at age 12, emerging knowledge about the developing adolescent brain suggests that decisions are more influenced by emotional states than previously acknowledged.[23] Specifically, the prefrontal cortex is a less developed control system, and the ventral striatum or reward system is less sensitive to small rewards in adolescents than in adults. Piker[22] and Grootens-Wiegers[23] suggest that "hot" decisions, those that are emotionally laden or driven by time pressure, benefit from more adult support. Decisions that are less emotionally charged, referred to as "cold" decisions, or those that have fewer long-term consequences and less time pressure, may need less adult support. This literature addresses research and treatment of chronic conditions, areas in which parental consent has traditionally been sought, and do not specifically address confidential care, where the mature minor doctrine has typically been applied.[15,24]

Some advocates for a more protective approach have applied advances in developmental neuroscience to the area of confidential care and are questioning a mature minor's capacity to consent.[25,26] Some advocates of confidential services also acknowledge that decision-making capacity is developing and uneven between ages 12 and 15.[15] Other advocates stress that youth who engage in sexual activity in early adolescence are more likely experiencing multiple effects of adverse childhood experiences[27] and that early sexual activity may itself be coerced or exploitative.[28] Confidential services can be a pathway to connect these particularly vulnerable early adolescents with supportive and protective care.[27] Nurses and other health care practitioners can maximize the decision-making capabilities of adolescents by making sure to give a full explanation of the alternative choices and exploring any possible coercion.[15]

ADOLESCENT RISK BEHAVIORS

The national Youth Risk Behavior Surveillance System (YRBSS) includes data from national, state, tribal, and large urban school district surveys of high school students conducted in the spring of odd-numbered years.[29] In the 2015 survey, the latest from which data are available, more than 29% of youth surveyed stated that they had felt so sad or hopeless during the 12 months before the survey that they had stopped some of their usual activities, with 17.7% seriously considering suicide.[30] More than 63% of high school students had had at least 1 drink of alcohol, and by 12th grade, 42.1% of students had drunk alcohol within the past 30 days. More than 41% of high school students report having had sexual intercourse, and by 12th grade, 58.1% of 12th graders overall and 57.2% of 12th grade girls had had sex,[30] 46.5% within the past 3 months. Use of alcohol, tobacco, and most drugs except for marijuana have decreased over time, following trends since 1991. Sexual activity has also slowly decreased over time, whereas the use of condoms and all forms of birth control have increased.[30] The prevalence of youth with at least 1 symptom of depression (29%) is concerning in the context of confidential care, because depression is linked to increased risk of unintended pregnancy in adolescents.[31]

Teen pregnancy is associated with lower educational attainments: almost a third of adolescent women who drop out of high school give pregnancy or parenting as a reason, and only 40% of adolescent mothers finish high school.[32] Adolescent pregnancy rates have been declining steadily since 1991 and were at their lowest point in 2016, at 20.3 births per 1000 female adolescents, compared with 61.8 births per 1000 in 1991.[33,34] An analysis of data from the National Survey of Family Growth showed that rates of sexual activity remained stable among teens between 2007 and 2012 and that declining pregnancy risk during this time was attributable to increased use of contraceptives.[35]

Rates of STIs are at an all-time high in the United States, however, with the highest rates of chlamydia and gonorrhea in the 15-year-old to 24-year old-age group.[36] Although syphilis rates are higher in young and older adults than in adolescents, they increased by 13% in adolescents from 2015 to 2016.[36] These statistics support both the success of and the need for greater access to services.

STATE STANDARDS FOR CONFIDENTIALITY

In general, the ability of adolescents to consent to a broad range of reproductive, mental health, and drug and alcohol services has increased over the past 30 years.[37] The only area of consent, however, on which all 50 states and the District of Columbia agree is in the diagnosis and treatment of STIs. Even in this area, 18 states allow a provider to notify the parents if the provider believes it is in the adolescent's best interest. In contrast, 26 states and the District of Columbia allow all minors ages 12 and older to consent to contraception, whereas 20 other states place restrictions, such as marriage, presence of a health condition, or determination of maturity.[37] For example, New York State allows all minors 12 and older to consent to contraception, STI services, prenatal care, adoption, and medical care for their own child and has no policy on abortion consent. Ohio has no policy on contraception, prenatal care, or medical care for a minor's own child; allows minor consent for STI services and adoption; and requires parental consent for abortion (**Table 2** for more information).

CONFIDENTIAL SERVICES AND PARENTAL NOTIFICATION

In a small survey of parents attending an adolescent clinic with their teens, parents could identify benefits of confidentiality.[38] They also wanted to be informed, however, about a wide range of topics, including depression, drug use, and sexual activity, even if their teen did not want them to know.[38] A retrospective study of primary care adolescent visits found that providers addressed more issues with teens, including not only sexual health and risk behaviors but also nutrition, diet, and exercise, if their parents were not in the room with the teen and provider for at least part of the visit.[39] In that study, only 46.5% of adolescents and 46% of parents reported that the teen spent time alone with a provider during their last visit.[39]

Multiple studies have highlighted the potential or actual change in utilization of confidential services when parental notification or consent is required. Reddy and colleagues[40] surveyed teens at Planned Parenthood clinics and found that 59% would stop using sexual health services, including STI testing, if parents were informed that they were seeking contraceptives. Only 1% of teens stated, however, that they would stop having sexual intercourse.[40] When Texas instituted parental notification for minors seeking abortions, the overall abortion rate of 15 year olds to 17 year olds declined 11% to 20%, but second-trimester abortion and birth rates increased.[41] Minors seeking

Table 2
State-by-state guides to minor consent and mandated reporting

Organization	Year of Publication	Specific Information	Web Site
Guttmacher Institute	Frequently updated	Minor consent for contraception, STI services, abortion, prenatal care, adoption, care of minor child	http://www.americaspromise.org/sites/default/files/d8/legacy/bodyfiles/teen-pregnancy-and-hs-dropout-print.pdf
Center for Adolescent Health & the Law	2010	Mature minor consent for general medical care	https://www.freelists.org/archives/hilac/02-2014/pdftRo8tw89mb.pdf
Child Welfare Information Gateway	2016 Updated every 2 years	Child abuse and neglect reporting, overview, includes reporting statutory rape and trafficking	https://www.childwelfare.gov/topics/systemwide/laws-policies/state/
Department of Health and Human Services (prepared by the Lewin Group)	2004	Statutory rape, detailed laws and reporting requirements	https://aspe.hhs.gov/system/files/pdf/75531/report.pdf

abortions in Illinois who were questioned about a potential parental notification law had generally negative views about this law, believing that the law would result in decreased access.[42] Recently, health economists compared YRBSS results in states with and without parental notification and found no change in sexual activity rates in states with parental notification. They did find, however, that teens in those states were more likely to use contraception than teens in states without required parental notification of family planning.[43] Because the YRBSS is based on self-report to a multiple-choice questionnaire, it is unclear if those teens were accessing Title X–funded clinics, which are exempt from state parental consent or notification laws (see below).

PUBLIC FUNDING AND CONFIDENTIALITY: TITLE X

The need for publicly funded contraceptive care has been growing since 2000, due to increased numbers of women in poverty.[44] Public funding for contraception and related health care has been available through Title X of the Public Health Service Act since 1970.[45] Women who earn up to 250% of the poverty line and all women under 20 are eligible for publicly funded contraception. The age specification is due to an assumption that young women under 20 are not able to access their parents' insurance due because of confidentiality concerns.[44] An estimated 1.1 million teens received contraceptive services at publicly funded clinics in 2013. Without these clinics, the estimated unintended pregnancy rate would have been 42% higher; without Title X clinics alone, the rate would have been 30% higher.[44]

When Title X was enacted, confidentiality and dignity were central to these regulations for all women and were made specifically available to all adolescents age 19 and younger in 1978.[46] Family participation in the care of adolescents was encouraged as long as confidentiality was protected. Consistent court decisions, in response to state or federal rulings since that time, have stated that adolescents must have access to Title X services without parental consent, even if parental consent is otherwise required by state law. The 1 exception to confidentiality protections, under Title X, is the mandated reporting of child abuse.[46]

Medicaid also protects the confidentiality of sexually active minors. The Health Insurance Portability and Accountability Act (HIPAA) recognizes that minors who can consent to confidential services have privacy rights to their confidential health records. Although HIPAA defers to state regulations, minors in states with parental consent or notification still have privacy rights to records for Title X services.[46] Prior to the current administration, clinics could only be prohibited from receiving Title X funding if they were unable to care for eligible patients. This regulation was recently overturned, in attempts to place additional restrictions on clinics seeking this funding. As this article goes to press, Title X funding remains in the FY 2018-2020 budget. However, specific allocations and mechanisms for grant application have not yet been determined. This may limit confidential services of reproductive health for adolescents in the 20 states that currently require parental consent.[37]

CONFIDENTIALITY AND MANDATORY REPORTING

Women's health practitioners working with adolescents must be cognizant of several overlapping regulations. In a setting that receives federal Title X funding, state mandatory child abuse reporting regulations may mandate reporting of consensual acts between disparate age minors or between minors and adults.[47,48] All 50 states have laws that mandate child abuse reporting, and federal minimum standards define child abuse as acts or failure to act by a parent or caretaker that result in "death, serious physical or emotional harm, sexual abuse, exploitation, or an imminent risk of serious harm."[49] States vary in their definitions of whether to report a reasonable suspicion that child abuse has occurred versus a suspicion that a child is at risk for abuse[49] (see **Table 2**).

There is also a great deal of variability in the specifics of sexual abuse reporting,[49] and the most controversial parts of these laws for nurses working in women's health are the state child abuse laws that mandate the reporting of statutory rape or the consensual relationships between disparate age minors or between minors and adults.[50–52] Many of these laws were revised starting in the 1990s, with the desired impact of lowering teen pregnancy rates by prosecuting adult men who were in relationships with adolescent minors.[53] There was also concern for protecting adolescents from coercive and abusive relationships with disparate age partners.[54] A more recent change to federal child abuse reporting law is the inclusion of sex trafficking as child abuse[49] and the introduction of safe harbor laws that encourage decriminalization of sexually exploited children and referrals to child protection agencies instead.[55] Although this is an important policy change, there are 2 concerns with this approach.[56] First, child welfare agencies may not be adequately resourced and oriented to protecting commercially sexually exploited children (CSEC), given that many CSEC are recruited by traffickers from the foster care system. Second, CSEC might avoid nurses and other health care practitioners because of mandatory reporting laws (see **Table 2**).

ELECTRONIC HEALTH RECORDS AND CONFIDENTIALITY

EHRs can help protect or inadvertently compromise adolescents' confidential information. A survey of Federally Qualified Health Centers (FQHCs) found that although most had written policies in place to protect adolescent confidentiality, only a few had separate medical records for confidential services. A minority of FQHCs had security blocks on medical records release or separate contact information in their EHRs for parents and adolescents.[57] Those who received Title X funding had more confidentiality protections in place for their records, highlighting the multiple ways in which Title X funding supports adolescent reproductive health. Under the Affordable Care Act, clinics are rewarded for showing meaningful use of an established government set of quality criteria in their EHRs.[58] This includes screening for chlamydia, depression, and substance use in adolescents.

Compliance with this requirement may inadvertently release information about these confidential services in the visit summary that is given to an adolescent and/or a parent.[59,60] Private insurance may release an explanation of benefits to parents about the minor or young adult child's use of confidential care; California recently enacted legislation that allows adolescents and young adults to receive this information directly.[60] Recommendations for providers who want to ensure adolescent confidentiality in the EHR include accurate knowledge of their state and Title X confidentiality laws; an understanding of their specific EHR functionality and careful attention to maximizing that functionality to avoid inadvertent releases of information in medical records, explanation of benefits, and meaningful use documents[60]; and use of a specific adolescent portal[59] (**Table 3**).

ADDITIONAL CONSIDERATIONS AND NURSING IMPLICATIONS

The history of health care in the United States has included deceptive, unethical, and coercive practices against poor and minority women and men.[61] Parents' relationship with health care providers may be marked by distrust, due to personal and historic

Table 3
Policies regarding electronic health records

Organization	Year of Publication
American College of Obstetricians and Gynecologists https://www.acog.org/Resources-And-Publications/Committee-Opinions/ Committee-on-Adolescent-Health-Care/Adolescent-Confidentiality-and- Electronic-Health-Records	2016
American Academy of Pediatrics http://pediatrics.aappublications.org/content/pediatrics/130/5/987.full.pdf	2012
Society for Adolescent Health and Medicine and American Academy of Pediatrics (electronic billing) http://pediatrics.aappublications.org/content/pediatrics/130/5/987.full.pdf	2016

experiences of racial discrimination,[62,63] which may make them more resistant to clinician assurances that they are providing high-quality care for their child. Ultimately this distrust may be passed to their adolescents. Immigrant families, many of whom have unauthorized family members,[64] may fear that any contacts with the health care system, including confidential care, would alert immigration officials.[65] Ongoing contact with diverse and culturally responsive health care providers, who are sensitive to power dynamics within their own institutions, may be able to bridge these historic and current chasms of distrust.[66] At the same time, nurses should advocate for policies that support confidential access[12] and guard against inadvertent breaches of confidentiality. This is imperative to ensure that adolescents have the full range of reproductive and health care options.

Confidential care highlights the transitions of adolescents toward adulthood and changes in parent-child relationships and as such can become the focus of conflict, when the underlying issue is often the transition itself.[67] Most parents support the concept of confidential communication between adolescents and health care providers, yet they are conflicted and unclear on the extent of confidentiality protections.[38,39] Nurses can aid this transition through anticipatory guidance,[6] active listening, and empathetic acknowledgment of parent and teen concerns, while maximizing adolescents' access to confidential care.

REFERENCES

1. World Health Organization. Ensuring human rights in the provision of contraceptive information and services. Geneva (Switzerland): World Health Organization; 2014.
2. United Nations Children's Fund (UNICEF). Convention on the Rights of the Child. n.d. Available at: http://www.ohchr.org/EN/ProfessionalInterest/Pages/CRC.aspx. Accessed June 13, 2009.
3. AAP Committee on Adolescence. Achieving quality health services for adolescents. Pediatrics 2016;138(2):e20161347.
4. Association of Women's Health, Obstetric & Neonatal Nursing. Confidentiality in Adolescent Health Care. J Obstet Gynecol Neonatal Nurs 2010;39(1):127–8.
5. Ford C, English A, Sigman G. Confidential health care for adolescents: position paper for the society for adolescent medicine. J Adolesc Health 2004;35(2):160–7.
6. Hagan J, Shaw J, Duncan P, editors. Bright futures: guidelines for health supervision of infants, children, and adolescents. 4th edition. Elk Grove Village (IL): American Academy of Pediatrics; 2017.

7. Schlam L, Wood JP. Informed consent to the medical treatment of minors: law and practice. Health Matrix Clevel 2000;10(2):141–74.
8. In re Gault, et al. In: US Supreme Court, editor. vol. 387 U.S. 1, Washington, DC, 1967.
9. English A, Bass L, Boyle AD, et al. State minor consent laws: a summary. 3rd edition. Chapel Hill (NC): Center for Adolescent Health and the Law; 2010. Available at: https://www.freelists.org/archives/hilac/02-2014/pdftRo8tw89mb.pdf. Accessed October 5, 2017.
10. Coleman DL, Rosoff PM. The legal authority of mature minors to consent to general medical treatment. Pediatrics 2013;131(4):786–93.
11. Maradiegue A. Minor's rights versus parental rights: review of legal issues in adolescent health care. J Midwifery Womens Health 2003;48(3):170–7.
12. Santa Maria D, Guilamo-Ramos V, Jemmott LS, et al. Nurses on the front lines: improving adolescent sexual and reproductive health across health care settings. Am J Nurs 2017;117(1):42–51.
13. Schapiro NA. Confidentiality and access to adolescent health care services. J Pediatr Health Care 2010;24(2):133–6.
14. Beauchamp TL, Childress JF. Principles of biomedical ethics. 7th edition. New York: Oxford University Press; 2013.
15. Steinberg L. Does recent research on adolescent brain development inform the mature minor doctrine? J Med Philos 2013;38(3):256–67.
16. Douglas J, Griswold V. Connecticut. In: US Supreme Court, editor. 381 U.S. 479, vol. 151. Washington, DC: Supreme Court; 1965. p. 481–6. Conn. 544, 200 A.2d 479, reversed.
17. Hein IM, De Vries MC, Troost PW, et al. Informed consent instead of assent is appropriate in children from the age of twelve: Policy implications of new findings on children's competence to consent to clinical research. BMC Med Ethics 2015;16(1):76.
18. Appelbaum PS, Grisso T. The MacArthur competence assessment tool for clinical research (MacCAT-CR). Sarasota (FL): Professional Resource Press; 2001.
19. Grisso T, Appelbaum PS, Hill-Fotouhi C. The MacCAT-T: a clinical tool to assess patients' capacities to make treatment decisions. Psychiatr Serv 1997;48(11):1415–9.
20. Hein IM, Troost PW, Lindeboom R, et al. Accuracy of the MacArthur competence assessment tool for clinical research (MacCAT-CR) for measuring children's competence to consent to clinical research. JAMA Pediatr 2014;168(12):1147–53.
21. Nelson LR, Stupiansky NW, Ott MA. The influence of age, health literacy, and affluence on adolescents' capacity to consent to research. J Empir Res Hum Res Ethics 2016;11(2):115–21.
22. Piker A. Balancing liberation and protection: a moderate approach to adolescent health care decision-making. Bioethics 2011;25(4):202–8.
23. Grootens-Wiegers P, Hein IM, van den Broek JM, et al. Medical decision-making in children and adolescents: developmental and neuroscientific aspects. BMC Pediatr 2017;17(1):120.
24. Alderman EM. Confidentiality in pediatric and adolescent gynecology: when we can, when we can't, and when we're challenged. J Pediatr Adolesc Gynecol 2017;30(2):176–83.
25. Barina R, Bishop JP. Maturing the minor, marginalizing the family: on the social construction of the mature minor. J Med Philos 2013;38(3):300–14.
26. Anderson JE. Brain development in adolescents: new research–implications for physicians and parents in regard to medical decision making. Issues Law Med 2015;30(2):193–6.

27. Sayegh A, Rose S, Schapiro NA. Condom availability in middle schools: evidence and recommendations. J Pediatr Health Care 2012;26(6):471–5.
28. Greenbaum J, Crawford-Jakubiak JE. Child sex trafficking and commercial sexual exploitation: health care needs of victims. Pediatrics 2015;135(3):566–74.
29. Brener ND, Kann L, Shanklin S, et al. Methodology of the youth risk behavior surveillance system. MMWR Recomm Rep 2004;53(RR-12):1–13.
30. Kann L, McManus T, Harris WA, et al. Youth risk behavior surveillance - United States, 2015. MMWR Surveill Summ 2016;65(6):1–174.
31. Hall KS, Richards JL, Harris KM. Social disparities in the relationship between depression and unintended pregnancy during adolescence and young adulthood. J Adolesc Health 2017;60(6):688–97.
32. Shuger L. Teen pregnancy & high school dropout: what communities can do to address these issues. Washington DC: The National Campaign to Prevent Teen and Unplanned Pregnancy and America's Promise Alliance; 2012.
33. Office of Adolescent Health. Trends in teen pregnancy and childbearing. 2016; Available at: https://www.hhs.gov/ash/oah/adolescent-development/reproductive-health-and-teen-pregnancy/teen-pregnancy-and-childbearing/trends/index.html. Accessed September 26, 2017.
34. Hamilton BE, Martin JA, Osterman MJK, et al. Births: provisional data for 2016. Hyattsville (MD): National Center for Health Statistics; 2017.
35. Lindberg L, Santelli J, Desai S. Understanding the decline in adolescent fertility in the United States, 2007–2012. J Adolesc Health 2016;59(5):577–83.
36. Centers for Disease Control and Prevention. Sexually transmitted disease surveillance 2016. Atlanta (GA): Centers for Disease Control and Prevention; 2017.
37. Guttmacher Institute. An overview of minors' consent law. State policies in brief 2017; Available at: https://www.guttmacher.org/print/state-policy/explore/over view-minors-consent-law. Accessed August 31, 2017.
38. Duncan RE, Vandeleur M, Derks A, et al. Confidentiality with adolescents in the medical setting: what do parents think? J Adolesc Health 2011;49(4):428–30.
39. Gilbert AL, Rickert VI, Aalsma MC. Clinical conversations about health: the impact of confidentiality in preventive adolescent care. J Adolesc Health 2014; 55(5):672–7.
40. Reddy DM, Fleming R, Swain C. Effect of mandatory parental notification on adolescent girls' use of sexual health care services. JAMA 2002;288(6):710–4.
41. Joyce T, Kaestner R, Colman S. Changes in abortions and births and the Texas parental notification law. N Engl J Med 2006;354(10):1031–8.
42. Kavanagh EK, Hasselbacher LA, Betham B, et al. Abortion-seeking minors' views on the Illinois parental notification law: a qualitative study. Perspect Sex Reprod Health 2012;44(3):159–66.
43. Sabia JJ, Anderson DM. The effect of parental involvement laws on teen birth control use. J Health Econ 2016;45:55–62.
44. Frost JJ, Frohwirth L, Zolna MR. Contraceptive needs and services, 2013 update. New York: Guttmacher Institute; 2015.
45. Napili A. Title X (Public Health Service Act) family planning program. Washington, DC: Congressional Research Service; 2017. RL-33644. p. 27.
46. English A. Adolescent confidentiality protections in Title X. National Family Planning and Reproductive Health Association; 2014. Available at: https://www.nationalfamilyplanning.org/document.doc?id=1559. Accessed September 27, 2017.
47. Glossner A, Gardiner K, Fishman M. Statutory rape: a guide to State laws and reporting requirements. Falls Church (VA): The Lewin Group; 2004.

48. Gudeman R, Monasterio E. Mandated child abuse reporting law: developing and implementing policies and trainings. Oakland (CA): National Center for Youth Law, National Family Planning Training Center; 2014.

49. Child Welfare Information Gateway. Definitions of child abuse and neglect: state statutes series. Child Welfare Information Gateway; 2016. Available at: https://www.childwelfare.gov/topics/systemwide/laws-policies/state/. Accessed September 5, 2017.

50. Miller C, Miller HL, Kenney L, et al. Issues in balancing teenage clients' confidentiality and reporting statutory rape among Kansas Title X clinic staff. Public Health Nurs 1999;16(5):329–36.

51. Sachs CJ, Weinberg E, Wheeler MW. Sexual assault nurse examiners' application of statutory rape reporting laws. J Emerg Nurs 2008;34(5):410–3.

52. Teare C, English A. Nursing practice and statutory rape. Effects of reporting and enforcement on access to care for adolescents. Nurs Clin North Am 2002;37(3): 393–404.

53. Donovan P. Can statutory rape laws be effective in preventing adolescent pregnancy? Fam Plann Perspect 1997;29(1):30–4, 40.

54. Kandakai TL, Smith LC. Denormalizing a historical problem: teen pregnancy, policy, and public health action. Am J Health Behav 2007;31(2):170–80.

55. Barnert ES, Abrams S, Azzi VF, et al. Identifying best practices for "Safe Harbor" legislation to protect child sex trafficking victims: decriminalization alone is not sufficient. Child Abuse Negl 2016;51:249–62.

56. English A. Mandatory reporting of human trafficking: potential benefits and risks of harm. AMA J Ethics 2017;19(1):54–62.

57. Beeson T, Mead KH, Wood S, et al. Privacy and confidentiality practices in adolescent family planning care at federally qualified health centers. Perspect Sex Reprod Health 2016;48(1):17–24.

58. EHR incentives & certification: Meaningful use definition & objectives. Health.gov 2015. 2017. Available at: https://www.healthit.gov/providers-professionals/meaningful-use-definition-objectives. Accessed October 1, 2017.

59. Thompson LA, Martinko T, Budd P, et al. Meaningful use of a confidential adolescent patient portal. J Adolesc Health 2016;58(2):134–40.

60. Williams RL, Taylor JF. Four steps to preserving adolescent confidentiality in an electronic health environment. Curr Opin Obstet Gynecol 2016;28(5):393–8.

61. Washington H. Medical apartheid: the dartk history of experimentation on black Americans from Colonial times to the present. New York: Random House; 2006.

62. Schwei RJ, Kadunc K, Nguyen AL, et al. Impact of sociodemographic factors and previous interactions with the health care system on institutional trust in three racial/ethnic groups. Patient Educ Couns 2014;96(3):333–8.

63. Armstrong K, Putt M, Halbert CH, et al. Prior experiences of racial discrimination and racial differences in health care system distrust. Med Care 2013;51(2): 144–50.

64. Clarke W, Turner K, Guzman L. One quarter of Hispanic children in the United States have an unauthorized immigrant parent. Bethesda (MD): National Research Center on Hispanic Children & Families; 2017.

65. Raymond-Flesch M, Siemons R, Pourat N, et al. "There is no help out there and if there is, it's really hard to find": a qualitative study of the health concerns and health care access of latino "DREAMers. J Adolesc Health 2014; 55(3):323–8.

66. Horn IB, Mitchell SJ, Wang J, et al. African-American parents' trust in their child's primary care provider. Acad Pediatr 2012;12(5):399–404.
67. Tebb K. Forging partnerships with parents while delivering adolescent confidential health services: a clinical paradox. J Adolesc Health 2011;49(4):335–6.

Integrating Optimal Screening, Intervention, and Referral for Postpartum Depression in Adolescents

Leigh Booth, EdD, RN*, Monika Wedgeworth, EdD, RN, CNE,
Adeline Turner

KEYWORDS

- Postpartum depression • Adolescents • Depression screening • Best practices

KEY POINTS

- Between 10% and 13% of women develop a mental disorder during the postpartum period.
- This percentage increased with adolescents and symptoms are commonly overlooked.
- These depressive disorders can be treated successfully if detected early, preventing more serious symptoms.
- The key is early recognition, screening, and intervention with an interprofessional approach.

According to the World Health Organization,[1] 10% to 13% of postpartum women develop a mental health disorder, most often depression, and this number is even higher in developing countries. The incidence of mental illness is higher in postpartum adolescents (ages 10–19 years of age), ranging from 26% to more than 50%. These percentages for postpartum depression (PPD) include women who miscarry or have abortions. Additionally, in adolescent women, symptoms are likely to be overlooked.[2] In 2015, the Centers for Disease Control and Prevention reported that 229,715 babies were born to adolescent mothers between the ages of 15 to 19.[2] This finding highlights the critical need for the early identification of PPD to decrease adverse outcomes associated with undetected and untreated depression.[3,4]

Disclosure Statement: There is no relationship with any commercial company that has a direct financial interest in subject matter or materials discussed in article or with a company making a competing product.
Capstone College of Nursing, The University of Alabama, 650 University Boulevard East, Tuscaloosa, AL 35401, USA
* Corresponding author.
E-mail address: labooth10@ua.edu

Nurs Clin N Am 53 (2018) 157–168
https://doi.org/10.1016/j.cnur.2018.01.003
0029-6465/18/© 2018 Elsevier Inc. All rights reserved.

nursing.theclinics.com

PPD can be treated successfully and, if detected early, treatment may prevent the development of more severe symptoms or negative outcomes. Nurse practitioners in primary care clinics are often on the front line of providing care to women during pregnancy and the postpartum period, emphasizing the importance of their role in the overall health and well-being of this high-risk population. The purpose of this article is to provide evidence-based best practices for early recognition and support of universal screening for PPD in adolescents. In addition, suggestions for the integration of behavioral health screenings into practice and recommendations for interprofessional collaboration are discussed.

BACKGROUND/SIGNIFICANCE

PPD, a devastating but manageable and treatable disease after pregnancy, often goes unrecognized. The effects permeate all aspects of a women's life, causing adverse effects on both mother and baby. These include worsening social support, impaired maternal–infant interactions, and delayed child development.[5] PPD is more common in adolescents owing to multiple age-specific stressors. Young mothers are often influenced by a lack of social support and high levels of social isolation.[2] Research reveals that adolescents with high levels of parental stress (stress brought on by the guardian of the teen parent) are more likely to experience PPD[6,7] and that adolescent parenting is often complicated by family dysfunction, emotional immaturity, life stress, and a lack of social support.[6,7]

PPD symptoms in an adolescent mother are associated with decreased maternal confidence in the ability to parent.[7] Interventions that target a reduction in the stress of parenting may lead to a lower depression severity in first-time adolescent mothers. Of particular importance is providing professional anticipatory guidance related to parenting stress and the use of coping mechanisms in high-risk groups.[7] Prenatal assessment of social support is one of the best ways to target interventions to treat and prevent PPD among adolescent mothers.[2]

Research supports screening for PPD in an open and nonjudgmental environment to reduce social stigma. This places primary care clinics at the forefront for early identification and referral to behavioral health treatment. The integration of PPD screening, with resultant positive outcomes, has been studied in relation care during postpartum obstetric visits, and by the pediatric practitioner for the mother during the baby's well-child appointments.[4,8,9] This method aids in identifying, treating, and referring adolescent women for behavioral health services. Therefore, given that adolescent mothers experience the highest rates and the most severe symptoms of PPD,[1,2] all adolescent mothers should be routinely screened for PPD during every interaction with a health care provider.

RISK FACTORS

Early identification of adolescents at risk for PPD may be complicated by the differences in risk factors and presenting symptoms of adolescent mothers compared with adult mothers.[2,6] Current screening instruments focus on predictive risk factors of general populations of pregnant women, using criteria such as marital status, pregnancy intention, obstetric complications, breastfeeding, and/or socioeconomic status indicators that are not targeted toward adolescents. Adolescent symptoms are more often influenced by social support and level of social isolation.[4] Additionally, in general, a combination of multiple factors for PPD place the adolescent at increased risk. These factors include negative life events (unplanned pregnancy or worsening of close relationships) and comorbid risk behaviors, such as substance abuse (ie, drinking or smoking before or during pregnancy), co-occurring psychiatric illness, and other stressors (help with care of infant or financial stressors).[4] Given the significantly higher risk of PPD in adolescents, nurses should be educated and aware of biological (ie, heredity and age) and nonbiological risk factors, as well as adolescent specific risk factors of PPD (**Box 1**).

PPD involves a range of moods that may vary in severity from day to day and is closely tied to perceived social support.[8] Often called, "the maternity blues," adolescents may present to the clinic with symptoms that are uncommon in adults and attributed to expected developmental adjustments. Depressed adolescents exhibit symptoms such as aggression, school absence, sexual promiscuity, and inappropriate expression of anger, and may run away from home.[10] Common red flags for depression in adolescents include a significant change in behavior, such as extroversion to introversion, or an adolescent who previously was a good student suddenly failing classes. The *Diagnostic and Statistical Manual of Mental Disorders,* 5th edition, diagnostic criteria for PPD is depression with a peripartum onset, which can occur as late as 4 weeks after childbirth. For women with onset of depression later than 4 weeks after delivery (after peripartum onset) are diagnosed as having major depressive disorder, with postpartum onset.[11,12]

PPD severity ranges from the baby blues to psychotic depression (presence of hallucinations or delusions, which may require hospitalization). Signs that may alert the

---

Box 1
Adolescent postpartum depression risk factors

Interpersonal factors

- Interpersonal functioning
  1. Depression before age 15

- Social
  1. Resides in a 1-parent household
  2. Lack of support from father of the baby
  3. Social isolation from peers
  4. Feelings of loneliness
  5. Perceived lack of social support

- Conflict among family members

Parenting and infant factors

- Lack of responsiveness and affection toward infant

- Unrealistic prenatal expectations of parenting
  1. Negative emotions when infant is crying
  2. Lack of family support
  3. High parenting stress

- Parenting beliefs
  1. Use of corporal or physical punishment
  2. Lack of empathy and negative regard for infant
  3. Potential for parent–child role reversal (as adolescent mother ages)

Other factors

- Generalized stress

- Negative self-esteem

Data from Kleiber BV, Dimidjian S. Postpartum depression among adolescent mothers: a comprehensive review of prevalence, course, correlates, consequences, and interventions. Clin Psychol Sci Prac 2014;21(1):48–66.

clinician during the visit include tearfulness, anxiety, and impaired concentration. The adolescent may express concern about her ability to care for the infant, or express feelings of guilt about wanting to be a normal teenager. Additionally, she may report somatic complaints such as excessive fatigue, changes in sleeping and/or eating habits, or nonspecific pain. Of particular concern is the adolescent presenting to the clinic with a lack of interest in the infant or a morbid fear that the infant might be harmed while in their care (**Box 2**).[2,6,12,13]

CASE STUDY

Amy is a 16-year-old girl who recently gave birth to her son Michael, a healthy baby boy. Before her pregnancy, Amy was involved in a variety of high school activities, including the dance and softball teams. During her pregnancy, she was temporarily released from both teams for medical reasons and has not been allowed to rejoin. Since Michael's birth, she has not returned to school and has been taking a few classes online to continue working toward her diploma.

Amy lost many friends during her pregnancy. The girls she considered to be her friends lost interest in her and stopped inviting her to afterschool activities. Her parents were unhappy about the unplanned pregnancy and are reluctant to be involved in Michael's care. Amy is still living with her parents and relies on them financially. To help with expenses, she has a part-time job. Michael's father is not involved, which places additional stress on Amy.

Today, Amy is at the clinic for her 6-week checkup. She arrives with her hair unwashed and in a messy ponytail. She is wearing a stained tee shirt and baggy pants. She complains of feeling tired all the time and states she has little appetite. She tearfully says, "The baby cries a lot and I can't seem to comfort him." The nurse

---

Box 2
Signs and symptoms of peripartum or postpartum depression

- Feelings of sadness or hopelessness
- Tearfulness
- Feeling overwhelmed
- Reduced interest in previous activities
- Feelings of worthlessness or guilt
- Anxiety, nervousness, or panic attacks
- Fear of inability to care for infant
- Excessive worry about infant
- Impaired concentration
- Irrational thinking
- Recurrent thoughts of harming self or infant
- Somatic complaints
  1. Appetite and/or weight changes
  2. Sleep changes
  3. Psychomotor agitation or retardation
  4. Fatigue/loss of energy
  5. Nonspecific pain

Data from Refs.[2,6,12,13]

practitioner completes a physical assessment and finds Amy to be physically healthy. She tells Amy that her feelings are characteristic of an adolescent mother facing the stressors of caring for her first child. The nurse practitioner advises Amy to nap when Michael naps and to eat her favorite foods. Amy leaves her appointment feeling discouraged and alone, and believes that no one understands her. As the weeks progress, she loses interest in her classes and eventually stops attending. She spends her free time in her room taking care of Michael with little social interaction.

POSTPARTUM DEPRESSION SCREENING

More than 50% of women with PPD are undiagnosed[14] and that percentage may be higher in adolescent mothers. In addition, suicide is a leading cause of death in postpartum women.[13] This risk is likely compounded when faced with a co-occurring mental illness and the stressful life circumstance of a teenage pregnancy. Given the long-term effects of PPD on families, the need for integrated behavioral health screenings and care in routine prenatal, postnatal, and well-child visits, it is critical to improve outcomes for infant, mother, and significant others.

The Association of Women's Health Obstetric and Neonatal Nurses recommends that primary care providers of women and newborns have routine screening protocols in place.[15] Additional screening recommendations are available from the American College of Obstetricians and Gynecologists,[16] the Department of Health and Human Services,[17] Agency for Healthcare Research and Quality (2013),[18] and the American Academy of Pediatrics.[19] These screening recommendations are summarized in **Table 1**.

In addition to screening guidelines, variability exists among depression screening tools recommended for use in primary care settings. The most common screening tools used in primary care practice environments include the Brief Patient Health Questionnaire-2 (PHQ-2), the PHQ-9, and the Edinburgh Postnatal Depression Scale.

Table 1
Summary of depression screening recommendations

Association of Women's Health, Obstetric and Neonatal Nurses[15]	Begins during prenatal care (early intervention) Continues after birth Staff trained to screen, educate, and refer Education and educational materials available Follow-up care arranged for positive results Emergency care as needed
American College of Obstetricians and Gynecologists[16]	Unclear recommendations of when and how often screening should occur Screening is strongly recommended Women with a history of depression need close monitoring Health care facilities should have follow-up in place for positive screening
Agency for Healthcare Research and Quality[18]	Screen from conception through end of first postnatal year Screen includes family history of depression Specifically screen at 4–6 wk, and 3–4 mo postpartum
American Academy of Pediatrics[19]	Screen mothers at well-child appointments for baby during the first year Edinburgh Postnatal Depression Scale for mothers at well-child visits at ages 2 wk, 2 mo, 4 mo, and 6 mo

Owing to its specificity for PPD, the EDPS (http://cope.org.au/health-professionals-3/perinatal-mental-health-disorders/calculating-score-epds/) is the most commonly used and validated tool in practice settings that focus on maternal and child health. The scale, developed in 1987[20] is a 10-item self-report questionnaire that has been translated into numerous languages. The American College of Obstetricians and Gynecologists has recently provided a recommendation highlighting the EDPS for screening:

> Routine and repeated screening for and treatment of mood disorders in pregnancy is recommended because of their increased rates in this population. The Edinburgh Postnatal Depression Scale administered in each trimester and postpartum, and more frequently if deemed necessary, is one option for such screening.[16]

The PHQ-2, a common brief screening measure used in many primary care settings, inquires about the extent to which an individual has experienced depressed mood or anhedonia over the previous 2 weeks. The PHQ-2 is only a screening measure. When the patient screens positive, the PHQ-9[20] must be administered. The PHQ-9 (**Fig. 1**) incorporates the first 2 questions of the PHQ-2, and is used to make the diagnosis of depression, because it includes the diagnostic criteria from the *Diagnostic and Statistical Manual of Mental Disorders,* 5th edition.

INTEGRATION OF BEHAVIORAL HEALTH SCREENING

For clinics to meet the goal of screening all adolescent mothers for PPD during routine visits, education and workflow redesign must occur to onboard all clinic staff about screening processes and procedures. The overarching integration goal is to improve patient outcomes by making PPD screening as familiar to nurses as recording patient vital signs. **Table 2** is an example of a 4-stage integration that includes stepped care for PPD. At each stage, the provider must make a clinical decision about whether further care is warranted, whether to proceed to the next stage of care, or if it is appropriate to disengage from the process. The assessment measures and clinical decision guidelines are specific to the screening tools used and are determined by the clinician.

Depending on the level of behavioral health integration (BHI) required, the treatment approach at the clinic may end with a brief intervention, such as patient education, and referral by the nurse practitioner to the behavioral health provider. Ideally, the level of BHI is such that the nurse practitioner is able to complete a transfer or "warm handoff" (introducing the adolescent mother directly to the behavioral health provider) after a positive screening for PPD. This step can take the form of a simple introduction to the behavioral health provider or by walking with her to make the behavioral health appointment with the scheduling clerk. This measure allows the adolescent mother to feel more secure knowing all her needs are being cared for at the clinic.

CONSEQUENCES OF UNTREATED POSTPARTUM DEPRESSION

Untreated PPD can have serious negative impacts on the adolescent mother's quality of life, as well as significant effects on the child (**Box 3**). The pervasive and toxic stress of PPD permeates all aspects of life, including social and intimate relationships, fetal growth and development, maternal–infant interactions, and poor child development through school age.[5,21] Adolescent mothers who are experiencing PPD may be reluctant to disclose these feelings to health care providers owing to the stigma associated

PATIENT HEALTH QUESTIONNAIRE-9 (PHQ-9)

Over the last 2 wk, how often have you been bothered by any of the following problems?
(Use "✔" to indicate your answer)

	Not at all	Several days	More than half the days	Nearly every day
1. Little interest or pleasure in doing things	0	1	2	3
2. Feeling down, depressed, or hopeless	0	1	2	3
3. Trouble falling or staying asleep, or sleeping too much	0	1	2	3
4. Feeling tired or having little energy	0	1	2	3
5. Poor appetite or overeating	0	1	2	3
6. Feeling bad about yourself — or that you are a failure or have let yourself or your family down	0	1	2	3
7. Trouble concentrating on things, such as reading the newspaper or watching television	0	1	2	3
8. Moving or speaking so slowly that other people could have noticed? Or the opposite — being so fidgety or restless that you have been moving around a lot more than usual	0	1	2	3
9. Thoughts that you would be better off dead or of hurting yourself in some way	0	1	2	3

FOR OFFICE CODING ___0___ + _____ + _____ + _____

=Total Score: _____

If you checked off **any** problems, how **difficult** have these problems made it for you to do your work, take care of things at home, or get along with other people?

Not difficult at all	**Somewhat difficult**	**Very difficult**	**Extremely difficult**
☐	☐	☐	☐

Fig. 1. The patient health questionnaire-9. (*Courtesy of* Drs Robert L. Spitzer, Janet B.W. Williams, Kurt Kroenke and colleagues, with an educational grant from Pfizer Inc. No permission required to reproduce, translate, display or distribute.)

with mental illnesses. In addition, there is a decreased likelihood of the mother attending pediatric visits or following provider recommendations.[6,22]

BEHAVIORAL HEALTH INTEGRATION

Primary care nurse led clinics are on the "front lines" of health care, providing inventive approaches to expanding and integrating services for increasingly complex

Table 2
Description of 4-stage process for identifying and implementing a scaled treatment approach to postpartum depression in primary care

Description of Activity	Provider
1. Collects prescreening data using single-item measures to identify individuals in need of further assessment	LPN, RN
2. Assesses patient health behaviors using standardized screening tool	Nurse practitioner
3. Engages patient with need for treatment in short conversation, provides feedback, education, and/or advice and referral to a behavioral health provider (as indicated)	Nurse practitioner
4. Provides brief therapy or additional treatment is screen indicates need for additional services	Behavioral health provider

populations.[8] This positions primary care providers to take the lead in the screening, brief treatment, and referral of adolescent mothers. Nurse-led clinics already serve women and children as primary care providers, and this factor is especially important in underserved and financially disadvantaged areas. However, as demonstrated by outdated treatment models, primary care and behavioral health care providers often operate in distinctly separate silos, with little sharing of information.[23]

Mental health conditions are increasingly common among patients seeking care at primary care clinics, and up to 70% of primary care visits may be attributed to psychosocial issues.[24] This number may be greater in higher risk populations, such as adolescents experiencing pregnancy and parenthood. The consensus among government agencies, researchers, and health care providers is that mental health and physical problems are interwoven.[17,25] A woman with PPD is not likely

---

Box 3
Summary of consequences of untreated postpartum depression

Adolescent mother
• Substance abuse
• Risk of pregnancy complications
• Smoking
• Poor interactions with infant
• Less likely to breastfeed
• Poor safety practices
• Increased risk for suicide/infanticide

Fetus/infant/child
• Low birth weight
• Irritability/crying
• Increased stress hormones
• Learning difficulties
• Delayed developmental milestones
• Aggression
• Poor social relationship development

Significant others
• Feelings of helplessness toward mother
• Increased depression in significant others
• Grief
• Intergenerational trauma owing to having a mother or significant other with untreated mental illness

Data from Refs.[2,6,13]

seek a mental health provider and this results in a significant treatment gap. In addition, co-occurring mental illness during pregnancy, such as depression, increases medical costs and contributes to poor outcomes.[4] Adolescents make up approximately 4% to 8% of depression diagnoses,[23] and the number of adolescents diagnosed with PPD is estimated to be nearly twice that of adult women.[4] Yet many new mothers remain undiagnosed. These data emphasize the need for screening and for behavioral health care integration into primary care for adolescents at risk for PPD.

Increasing national focus on integrated care has led primary care clinics to begin to offer BHI and to serve as comprehensive sites for patient care.[17,25] Federal agencies such as Substance Abuse and Mental Health Services Administration and Health Resources and Services Administration have strongly emphasized integrated behavioral health as the new model of practice for primary care visits.[17,25] Integrated care allows patients to access both physical and mental health services in their own communities, allowing for mental health promotion, as well as for monitoring and managing mental health conditions. This approach to services can be accomplished by a variety of levels of integration, from brief screening and referral, to fully integrated behavioral health collaboration. There are several models of behavioral health and primary care integration. **Table 3** illustrates the 3 basic distinctions among integration types.

Integrating behavioral health at the most basic level of collaborative care requires more than initiation of simple screening, brief treatment, and referral. Clinical practice changes that affect routines are often difficult to initiate owing to existing workloads

Table 3
Collaborative care categorizations at a glance

Coordinated	Colocated	Integrated
Routine screening for behavioral health problems conducted in primary care setting	Medical and behavioral health services located in same facility	Medical and behavioral health services located in same facility or separate locations, with close collaboration
Referral relationship between primary care and behavioral health	Referral process for medical cases to be seen by behavioral specialists	One treatment plan with behavioral and medical elements
Routine exchange of information between both settings	Enhanced informal communication between providers owing to proximity	Team works together to deliver care, using prearranged protocol
Primary care provider delivers behavioral health interventions using brief algorithms	Consultation between the providers increases skills of both groups	Team composed of physician and $\geq$1 other—physician's assistant, nurse practitioner, nurse, case manager, family advocate, behavioral health therapist
Referrals to community	Increase level and quality of behavioral health services; significant reduction in missed appointments	Use of database to track care

From Collins C, Hewson DL, Munger R, et al. Evolving models of behavioral health integration in primary care. New York: Milbank Memorial Fund; 2010. p. 504; with permission.

and time constraints of visits. Clinic staff must be trained on all aspects of new processes, including the overall benefits of BHI (decreased health care costs, holistic patient-centered care), alteration of visit workflow, appropriate use of screening tool(s), brief treatment, documentation, referral, and follow-up.[23] Clinic directors must be proactive in seeking assistance and resources to assist primary care providers with effective BHI.

CASE STUDY ALTERNATE ENDING

The nurse practitioner observes signs and symptoms in Amy, and believes that additional steps should be taken to assess her mental symptoms. The nurse practitioner choses a standardized screening tool to assess Amy. Among other things, the Edinburgh Postnatal Depression Scale assessed how Amy is feeling and how much she has laughed lately. The criteria for further evaluation for depression is a score of more than 10 and Amy scores a 15. The nurse practitioner explains to Amy that these feelings can be treated, and provides her with information about treatment options. A referral is made to a behavioral health provider to further assess her depressive symptoms and provide treatment as indicated.

Six weeks later, Amy returns and feels much better. She has returned to school and is thriving. She also reports that she is really enjoying her baby, and is participating in a local teen mom support group where she made new friends.

SUMMARY

PPD in adolescents is a complex issue with far-reaching and long-lasting consequences to the mother, infant, significant other, and family. Early intervention and treatment cannot be accomplished without the integration of screening (and treatment) for PPD in primary care settings, where high-risk adolescents seek health care. Validated tools are successful in well-child and obstetric settings; however, they are not currently well-integrated into many care environments. Adolescents are at particularly high-risk for PPD and the associated complications; therefore, adolescent mothers should be screened for PPD at each health care interaction for the entire first year after pregnancy. Ideally behavioral health treatment begins immediately; however, processes should be put in place at clinics to integrate behavioral health at a variety of levels to better serve this group.

REFERENCES

1. World Health Organization (WHO). Maternal mental health. 2017. Available at: http://www.who.int/mental_health/maternal-child/maternal_mental_health/en/2017. Accessed September 15, 2017.
2. Nunes AP, Phipps MG. Postpartum depression in adolescent and adult mothers: comparing prenatal risk factors and predictive models. Matern Child Health J 2013;17(6):1071–9.
3. Centers for Disease Control and Prevention (CDC). Depression among women. 2017. Available at: https://www.cdc.gov/reproductivehealth/depression/index.htm. Accessed September 15, 2017.
4. Mgonja S, Schoening A. Postpartum depression screening at well-child appointments: a quality improvement project. J Pediatr Health Care 2017;31(2):178–83.

5. McDonald S, Wall J, Forbes K, et al. Development of a prenatal psychosocial screening tool for post-partum depression and anxiety. Paediatr Perinat Epidemiol 2012;26(4):316–27.
6. Kleiber BV, Dimidjian S. Postpartum depression among adolescent mothers: a comprehensive review of prevalence, course, correlates, consequences, and interventions. Clin Psychol Sci Pract 2014;21(1):48–66.
7. Venkatesh KK, Phipps MG, Triche EW, et al. The relationship between parental stress and postpartum depression among adolescent mothers enrolled in a randomized controlled prevention trial. Matern Child Health J 2014;18(6):1532–9.
8. Chen H, Wang J, Ch'ng YC, et al. Identifying mothers with postpartum depression early: integrating perinatal mental health care into the obstetric setting. ISRN Obstet Gynecol 2011. https://doi.org/10.5402/2011/309189.
9. Yogman MW. Postpartum depression screening by pediatricians: time to close the gap. J Dev Behav Pediatr 2016;37(2):157.
10. Townsend M, Morgan K. Essentials of psychiatric mental health nursing: concepts of care in evidence-based practice. Philadelphia: F.A Davis; 2017. p. 7.
11. Segre L, Davis W. Postpartum depression and perinatal mood disorder in the DSM. 2013. Available at: www.postpartum.net/wp-content/uploads/2014/11/DSM-5-Summary-PSI.pd. Accessed September 25, 2017.
12. American Psychiatric Association. Diagnostic and statistical manual of mental disorders: DSM-5. Arlington (VA): American Psychiatric Publishing; 2013.
13. Roy-Byrne PP. Postpartum blues and unipolar depression: epidemiology, clinical features, assessment, and diagnosis. In: UpToDate, Post TW, editors. Waltham (MA): UpToDate; 2014.
14. Myers ER, Aubuchon-Endsley N, Bastian LA, et al. Efficacy and safety of screening for postpartum depression. Rockville (MD): Agency for Healthcare Research and Quality; 2013.
15. Association of Women's Health, Obstetrics, and Neonatal Nurses: position statement. Mood and anxiety disorders in pregnant and postpartum women. J Obstet Gynecol Neonatal Nurs 2015;44(5):687–9.
16. Fleming N, O'Driscoll T, Becker G, et al. Adolescent pregnancy guidelines. J Obstet Gynaecol Can 2015;37(8):740–56.
17. US Department of Health and Human Services. United States Department of Health and Human Services: healthy people 2010: understanding and improving health. Washington, DC: US Government Printing Office; 2000. p. 15–20.
18. Agency for Healthcare Research and Quality (AHRQ). Efficacy and safety of screening for postpartum depression. 2013. Available at: https://www.ahrq.gov/research/findings/postpartumdep.html. Accessed September 12, 2017.
19. American Academy of Pediatrics (AAP). Maternal depression screening. 2016. Available at: https://www.aap.org/en-us/advocacy-and-policy/state-advocacy/documents/maternaldepressionscreeningguidance.pdf. Accessed September 12, 2017.
20. PHQ-9. Developed by Drs Robert L. Spitzer, Janet B.W. Williams, Kurt Kroenke and colleagues, with an educational grant from Pfizer Inc. No permission required to reproduce, translate, display or distribute.
21. Liu Y, Kaaya S, Chai J, et al. Maternal depressive symptoms and early childhood cognitive development: a meta-analysis. Psychol Med 2017;47(4):680–9.
22. Figueiredo B, Bifulco A, Pacheco A, et al. Teenage pregnancy, attachment style, and depression: a comparison of teenage and adult pregnant women in a Portuguese series. Attach Hum Dev 2006;8(2):123–38.

23. Collins C, Hewson DL, Munger R, et al. Evolving models of behavioral health integration in primary care. New York: Milbank Memorial Fund; 2010. p. 504.
24. Robinson P, Reiter J. Behavioral consultation and primary care. Switzerland: Springer Science+ Business Media, LLC; 2007.
25. Substance Abuse and Mental Health Services Administration (SAMHSA). Health Care and Health Systems Integration. 2017. Available at: https://www.samhsa.gov/health-care-health-systems-integration. Accessed September 22, 2017.

Section III: Common to Childbearing Aged Women

Preconception Care for the Patient and Family

Elizabeth Hall, RN, APRN, DNP, WHNP-BC, SANE*, Robingale Panepinto, RN, DNP, FNP,
Elizabeth Keeley Bowman, RN, DNP, WHNP

KEYWORDS

- Preconception • Planning • Pregnant • Prenatal guidelines

KEY POINTS

- Holistic preconception counseling is essential for childbearing age patients.
- A cocreated preconception plan optimizes birth outcomes.
- It is important to promote health options, assess risk factors and referral needs.

INTRODUCTION

Preconception counseling (PCC) is important for women of childbearing age and their family members as they plan to manage pregnancy and anticipate outcomes. In many ways, the United States is an international leader of health care but there is still room for improved pregnancy outcomes. Women who have a decreased awareness and knowledge of the importance of preconception health are more likely to demonstrate poor adherence to preconception care recommendations.[1] Two concerning poor pregnancy outcomes are low birthweight and preterm births. Preterm birth rates are trending in the right direction but even with a 7-year decline the rate was ll.39% in 2013, and yet the low birthweight has been steady at 8.02%.[2] Health care providers using reflective practice are key when promoting optimal pregnancy outcomes for women and family members.[3] Combining the woman's prior medical history and her family genetics pattern, along with the partner's genetics, assists in illuminating high-risk concerns that need to be addressed during the preconception period.

Reflective practice is an awareness of being present in the moment and using insight gained from previous similar experiences to respond to patients and families.[3] There are several fruits of reflective practice that evolve over time through reflection on past experiences. Mindfulness and poise are 2 attributes that connect the patient and provider because the provider is seen as being available. As the practitioner uses

Disclosure Statement: None.
Vanderbilt University School of Nursing, 461 21st Avenue South, Nashville, TN 37240, USA
* Corresponding author.
E-mail address: Elizabeth.d.hall@vanderbilt.edu

mindfulness, viewing reality as it is, the moment between the patient, practitioner, and family becomes self-affirming and less cumbersome.[3] Poise, how well one knows one's self, is important for the practitioner to best frame the relationship during the process of developing rapport with the patient.[3] The patient seeking PCC may feel vulnerable, and the practitioner can use reflective practice to establish the supportive rapport needed to cocreate a patient-centered plan for pregnancy. By using reflective practice, the patient, family, and provider experience feelings of self-worth, being valued, and are empowered to engage in the encounter. Thus, any negative energy potentially can be converted to positive energy with each response of the unfolding encounter.[3]

A primary part of the PCC encounter, preconception health education includes the woman in creating her action plan to be healthy before, during, and after pregnancy. Providers using reflective practice incorporate mindfulness and poise to create a plan with the woman and her family. Reflective practice supports and eases the woman's transition from the contemplation to the action stage of Prochaska's transtheoretical model (TTM).[3,4] The TTM is a model that stages the behavior change process through preparation and realization, which supports proactive health decisions by educating and encouraging the patient. These stages are experienced as a patient proceeds with her pregnancy plans. The TTM addresses emotions, cognition, and behaviors in a stage-based process of health behavior change that is essential to consider in relation to the nature and timing of PCC with patients.[4] There are 6 stages of change: precontemplation, contemplation, preparation, action, maintenance, and termination.

PRECONCEPTION PLANNING

The counseling consists of 5 main areas of focus that the provider should address with the woman and her family during the preconception encounter: history, physical assessment, laboratory evaluation, genetic counseling, and health promotion[5] (Fig. 1). By addressing these health areas, the likelihood for improved outcomes is increased for the mother and fetus.[1,6]

Counseling begins when the woman contacts the office for an appointment. The appointment scheduler should ask the woman to make a list of questions to bring for discussion at the PCC appointment. This first appointment is a vital time for the provider to develop rapport with the woman, which may result in an increased potential for adherence, as well as the likelihood of an optimal outcome.

ENCOUNTER

Once the appointment is scheduled and the woman arrives for the consultation, the provider has an opportunity to engage her in a holistic approach using reflective practice.[3] The following are included in the encounter:

- Establish a strong patient–provider rapport through active listening, asking open-ended questions, addressing goals, and inquiring about care preferences. What are her expectations? What is her family structure and what are their goals?
- Frame the interview to address her questions and expectations. Set up an opportunity within the interview to discuss the timeline for conception, and focus on her personal plans.
- Offer information addressing physical, emotional, and spiritual care.

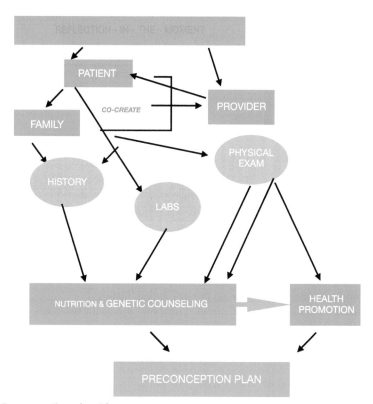

Fig. 1. Preconception algorithm.

The provider should focus the encounter on the woman's personal plans. Incorporating reflective practice in the moment provides acknowledgment and encourages the woman and her family to share pregnancy goals and questions.

HISTORY

The history interview includes an inquiry of maternal medical history and an obstetric risk assessment of the mother's and the father's families (**Table 1**). The provider should ask about the patient's perceived existing support systems, personal lifestyle choices, emotional needs, and spiritual preferences that enhance her feelings of well-being. When the provider and the woman consider these preferences, the cocreated PCC plan is optimized. This interaction is an opportunity to further strengthen rapport with the woman and her family, and to identify a functional support network at the beginning of the preconception phase.[3,5] Included in the history interview are

Maternal and family medical history
- Personal health history
- Mental health: depression, anxiety, eating disorders, bipolar mental illness, prior postpartum depression
- Chronic disease processes: diabetes, thrombocytopenia, hypertension
- Genetic or autoimmune disease processes: autoimmune- rheumatoid arthritis, systemic lupus erythematosus, systemic sclerosis (scleroderma), autoimmune

Table 1
Comprehensive preconception patient history

History	Variable Attributes and Factors
Medical History (including gynecological)	Menstrual, sexual, sexually transmitted infections (STIs), immunizations, varicella, herpes simplex virus (HSV), contraception (current and past)
Obstetric History	Vaginal birth after cesarean (VBAC) or trial of labor after cesarean (TOLAC)
Family and Genetic History	History of genetic diseases (eg, Tay Sachs, sickle cell anemia, cystic fibrosis; see **Table 4**)
Psychosocial History	Tobacco, alcohol, drugs, depression, domestic violence, and employment setting for risks and nutrition
Environment and Infectious Disease Exposure	Cytomegalovirus (CMV), toxoplasmosis, household lead

thyroid disease (Hashimoto and Graves disease), type I diabetes mellitus, clotting-factor V Leiden, and prothrombin mutations (**Table 2**)
- Cancer

Paternal medical history and paternal family medical history
- Life experiences (alcohol and street drugs) and medical treatments can reduce the number of sperm
- Toxic substance exposure can increase male infertility and increases the incidence of diseases during all stages of life for unconceived child
- Increased risk for low birthweight of newborns by 20% from secondhand smoke
- Screen men for sexually transmitted infections.[7]

PRECONCEPTION PHYSICAL ASSESSMENT

Before conception, providers need to perform a thorough physical assessment, as well as order pertinent laboratory tests. Each woman is different and the provider must use sound clinical judgment to establish what additional assessments are needed. **Table 3** includes assessment recommendations, as well as findings that are of concern.[8]

PRECONCEPTION LABORATORY ASSESSMENT

Providers should obtain the necessary laboratory examinations as indicated by the current health status of the woman. In addition, consider any other conditions that could affect current fertility and the subsequent pregnancy (**Table 4**.)[8]

Table 2
Maternal and paternal family history

Disease	Referral Recommended
Sickle Cell	African American patients
Tay Sachs	Ashkenazi Jewish, French Canadian patients
Thalassemia	Mediterranean, African, Asian, Middle Eastern patients (depending on type of Thalassemia and family history)
Cystic Fibrosis	White men of northern European descent
Hemophilia	Maternal or paternal family history
Duchenne muscular dystrophy	Maternal or paternal family history

Table 3
Physical assessment

Test	Considerations
Blood Pressure	Elevated before pregnancy increases the risk of maternal or fetal complications during pregnancy, including preeclampsia and eclampsia
Body Mass Index (BMI)	Obesity affects fertility and increases the risk of pregnancy complications
Heart	Maternal cardiac structural and electrical abnormalities, including murmurs and arrhythmias, may exacerbate and become life-threatening during pregnancy
Breasts	Assess for lumps and/or masses, perform mammogram per guidelines, assess for potential breastfeeding issues
Thyroid	Check for masses, enlargement, and hormone levels; altered thyroid function affects fertility and pregnancy
Abdomen	Check for tenderness and masses
Mouth	Check for caries and gum inflammation; increased risk of systemic infection
Genital tract	Papanicolaou (Pap) smear per guidelines, bimanual examination, STI testing

Data from Chames MC. Prenatal care. University of Michigan, Quality Department. Available at: http://www.med.umich.edu/1info/FHP/practiceguides/newpnc/PNC.pdf. Accessed October 2, 2017.

GENETIC COUNSELING REFERRAL

The results of the history and physical, as well as laboratory reports, may indicate the need for referral. Referral for additional testing and genetic counseling depend on findings related to several factors, such as family history, the woman's medical history, obstetric history, paternal family, or personal medical history.[9]

HEALTH PROMOTION

PCC provides an opportune time to address health promotion before pregnancy (**Box 1**). Encourage healthy behaviors, including prenatal vitamins, calcium, folic acid, exercise, and so forth.

Preconception Nutritional Needs

Prenatal vitamin use, in addition to a healthy diet containing vitamins and minerals, is beneficial to a healthy pregnancy and newborn. Studies show prenatal vitamins containing folic acid, calcium, iron, and vitamin D contribute to prevention of serious health effects to the mother and newborn. Folic acid influences healthy neural tube development and prevention of brain and spinal cord defects. Calcium and vitamin D are beneficial for a baby's bone development and, although a mother's healthy diet may supply these, additional amounts may be needed and recommended by the provider. Iron prevents anemia in the mother and promotes growth and development of the baby. Suggested best practice is to take prenatal vitamins are during the preconception period and throughout the pregnancy and breastfeeding period. In addition, the provider may advise additional dosage of a particular mineral and or vitamin to enhance a healthy pregnancy and baby. Findings noted in the *British Journal of Nutrition* 2016 research review, suggest iron supplementation of infants may influence their subsequent psychomotor development.[10]

Table 4
Routine and suggested laboratory examinations

Laboratory Examinations	Considerations
STIs	Certain STIs may affect fertility due to scarring; medications used to treat infection must be evaluated related to safety of use during pregnancy
Rubella immunity status	Immunity status before pregnancy must be determined and immunization should completed whenever possible before conception because immunization is contraindicated during pregnancy
Varicella immunity status	See rubella
Tuberculosis (TB) skin test	Test high-risk women (health care workers, arrived from or traveled to countries with high TB prevalence) because treatment can be dangerous during pregnancy
Genetic testing	Based on medical, gynecologic, or obstetric history, and family history of both parents
Glycosylated hemoglobin (Hgb A1C)	If indicated, determine glycemic control; good control can limit risk to fetus
Initial type 2 diabetes assessment	Women with high BMI, hypertension, or high cholesterol, as well as those older than 40 years need an initial screening
Phenylalanine (PKU) level	Known or suspected PKU
Lead levels	If at risk for exposure
CMV	Controversial; useful if woman works around young children (daycare age), has a child in daycare, or has possible work exposure
Toxoplasmosis	Controversial; useful if the woman has a risk of exposure (dietary, exposure to cats, exposure at work)
Influenza	Vaccine must be administered before pregnancy or early in pregnancy

Data from Chames MC. Prenatal care. University of Michigan, Quality Department. Available at: http://www.med.umich.edu/1info/FHP/practiceguides/newpnc/PNC.pdf.

Risk Factors

Discuss risk factor reduction, including alcohol, smoking, environmental feline litter box for cats residing outside or inside, substance abuse, stress, and coping. Also, this discussion should include

Box 1
Preconception health and wellness promotion

Health and wellness promotion activities

Review test results, if available, and dating criteria

Expected weight gain in pregnancy

Breastfeeding

Obesity counseling (nutrition and exercise)

Substance use

Sexual behaviors

Table 5 Preconception care for patient and family		
Background Issues	**Screening Examinations**	**Wellness Education**
History and physical examination	Blood type and antibody screen	Education and planning (genetic counseling, health promotion)
Medical history (menstrual, sexual, immunizations, varicella, HSV, contraception)	Hemoglobin, hematocrit, platelet count	Counsel on significant positive findings elicited by history, physical, or test results; review test results
Varicella titer		
Obstetric history	Rubella titer	
Family and genetic history	Hepatitis B surface antigen	Screening for aneuploidy
Psychosocial history (tobacco, alcohol, drugs, depression, domestic violence, employment, and nutrition)	HIV; STI screening (gonorrhea, chlamydia, syphilis)	Nutrition in pregnancy (folate, calcium, fish, listeria); expected weight gain
Urine culture, pap smear, genetic screening, diabetes testing		Breastfeeding
Environment and infectious disease exposure (CMV, toxoplasmosis, lead)	Hepatitis C testing, TB testing	Obesity counseling
Influenza vaccination		VBAC or TOLAC
Complete physical examination (height, weight, BMI, blood pressure, pelvic examination)	First trimester screening	Discuss referral for genetic counseling if needed
		Discuss need for referral to high risk

- Reviewing fetal risk, including optimal blood glucose for at least 3 months before pregnancy in women with diabetes
- Anticipatory guidance for what the woman should expect in caring for herself physically, emotionally, and culturally
- Referral potential: as needed and individually based.

SUMMARY

Holistic PCC requires attention to all aspects of the woman and her prospective family unit. **Table 5** provides a quick reference to remind providers of the essentials of PCC. When the provider uses a holistic approach combined with reflective practice, the woman will be empowered through knowledge and awareness. Provider support and guidance, and needed screenings, begin during the PCC to promote optimal mother and fetal outcomes. The established rapport between the provider and the woman promotes adherence with pregnancy health recommendations.

The PCC appointment focuses on gathering a thorough history, performing physical and bimanual examinations, Papanicolaou (Pap) screening, and obtaining serum for several laboratory diagnostic examinations. In addition, a genetic counseling discussion based on identified issues during the visit may be warranted. This approach also provides health promotion education related to how the patient can live healthy and addresses issues of high priority when establishing positive patient pregnancy goals.

REFERENCES

1. Goodfellow A, Frank J, McAteer J, et al. Improving preconception health and care: a situation analysis. BMC Health Serv Res 2017;17(1):595.
2. Centers for Disease Control. "CDC National Vital Statistics Reports" Available at: cdc.gov/nchs/data_access/Vitalstatsonline.htm. Accessed October 2, 2017.

3. Johns C. Exploring reflection. Being available. Becoming a reflective practitioner. John Wiley & Sons; 2009. p. 9–12, 115.

4. Prochaska JO, Velicer WF. The transtheoretical model of health behavior change. Am J Health Promot 1997;12(1):38–48.

5. Chames MC, et al. "Prenatal care." Available at: http://www.med.umich.edu/1info/FHP/practiceguides/newpnc/PNC.pdf. Accessed October 2, 2017.

6. Centers for Disease Control. "Show your love: steps to a healthier me and baby-to-be." Available at: cdc.gov/preconception/showyourlove/documents/Healthier Baby Me Plan.pdf. Accessed 2 October 2017.

7. Centers for Disease Control. "Preconception health and health care: information for men." Available at: cdc.gov/preconception/men.html. Accessed October 2, 2017.

8. Sackey, Joyce A. "The preconception visit." UpToDate. http://www.uptodate.com. ckmproxy.mc.vanderbilt.edu/contents/the-preconception-office-visit?source=search_result&search=preconception%20counseling&selectedTitle=1~89. Accessed September 24, 2017.

9. American College of Obstetricians and Gynecologists. "Screening and diagnostic testing for genetic disorders" Available at: www.acog.org/-/media/For-Patients/Screening-and-Diagnostic-Testing-for-Genetic-Disorders.pdf?dmc=1&ts=20170924T0303345151. Accessed September 24, 2017.

10. Chmielewska A, Dziechciarz P, Gieruszczak-Białek D, et al. Effects of prenatal and/or postnatal supplementation with iron, PUFA or folic acid on neurodevelopment: update. Br J Nutr 2016. https://doi.org/10.1017/S0007114514004243.

Intimate Partner Violence
What Health Care Providers Should Know

Anne McKibbin, PhD, RN[a],*, Kathy Gill-Hopple, PhD, RN, SANE-A, SANE-P[b]

KEYWORDS

- Intimate partner violence • Screening • Abuse • Domestic violence
- Medical documentation

KEY POINTS

- Intimate partner violence (IPV) is a health epidemic. Health care professionals have a unique and critical role to play.
- The Centers for Disease Control and Prevention describes IPV as "physical violence, sexual violence, stalking and psychological aggression (including coercive acts) by a current or former intimate partner."
- IPV screening tools are useful for detecting violence and developing intervention strategies to prevent future harm.
- Health care providers need information related to state laws, accurate documentation skills, and knowledge of national and local resources to effectively serve women who have been exposed to IPV.

INTRODUCTION

Intimate partner violence (IPV) is a public health epidemic affecting 1 in every 4 women.[1] This adversely affects health and, in the United States, costs $8.3 billion each year.[2] Health care professionals have a unique and critical role in the identification and treatment of women exposed to IPV. Often, women who are exposed to acts of IPV do not disclose the abuse based on many factors such as fear and confusion related to what they have experienced. When conducted face-to-face, both routine and repeated screenings have the potential to markedly increase the identification of IPV because a woman's abuse status can change over time. This article briefly reviews the standard of practice for health care professionals, so they can engage in an informed response to IPV, which is crucial to the safety of the woman, can improve health outcomes, and prevent further violence.

[a] Tuscaloosa County Domestic Violence Task Force, 2204 University Boulevard, Tuscaloosa, AL 35401, USA; [b] Forensic Nursing Services, Medical University of South Carolina, 169 Ashley Avenue, Charleston, SC 29401, USA
* Corresponding author.
E-mail address: aemckibbin1@gmail.com

Nurs Clin N Am 53 (2018) 177–188
https://doi.org/10.1016/j.cnur.2018.01.007
0029-6465/18/© 2018 Elsevier Inc. All rights reserved.

INTIMATE PARTNER VIOLENCE DEFINED

IPV, as defined by the Centers for Disease Control and Prevention, is "physical violence, sexual violence, stalking and psychological aggression (including coercive acts) by a current or former intimate partner. An intimate partner is a person with whom one has a close personal relationship."[3] This violence is a pattern of controlling, assaultive, and/or coercive behavior against an intimate partner.[4] Behaviors of the abuser may include physical, sexual, psychological, and economic coercion or abuse.[5] The abuse can occur in a variety of relationships: married, separated, divorced, dating, heterosexual, or same-sex couples. It does not depend on sexual intimacy.[3]

The statistics on IPV are staggering. According to the National Coalition Against Domestic Violence, in the United States there are more than 10 million victims of IPV.[1] In cases in which a firearm is present during the abuse, there is a significant increase in the risk of homicide.[1] IPV is the most common cause of injury in women aged 18 to 44 years and is associated with numerous medical and health conditions for victims and their children.[6] Unfortunately, very few individuals (about 34%) seek medical care for their injuries following an abusive event.[1] To improve response efforts for victims of IPV, health care professionals should take the time to adhere to recommendations for screening, increase their knowledge of abuse indicators, supportive care, safety planning, documentation, and awareness of community resources and referral processes.

SCREENING FOR INTIMATE PARTNER VIOLENCE

Screening tools for IPV are useful for detecting violence and developing intervention strategies for preventing future harm. The US Preventive Services Task Force recommends clinicians screen women of childbearing ages and provides resources or refers women who screen positive to intervention services.[7] The task force concluded that screening protocols for elderly women are limited based on the absence of standards.[7]

Screening and counseling for IPV without a copayment or coinsurance when delivered by a network provider is a core service included in the preventive care policy of the Affordable Care Act.[8] To fulfill this requirement, health care professionals must have a safe and effective system in place for screening women for IPV. Minimum requirements of preventive care screening include that health care providers perform an IPV assessment on female patients 12 years of age and older.[9]

Despite the availability of screening tools, the frequency of screening varies across health care disciplines and environments. This may be due to a lack of curricular inclusion. A report detailing health professionals' educational preparation for treating IPV indicated that, in schools and colleges of medicine, dentistry, and public health, more attention should be placed on the screening, identification, health problems, interventions, and professional competencies required for addressing violence and abuse. In contrast, schools of nursing have made the most significant progress in curriculum development related to IPV.[10]

Setting

The setting for conducting IPV screening must be carefully considered. The first consideration is to provide a safe and confidential location that fosters a setting in which the woman is able to disclose exposure to violence. Screening should take place with the woman fully dressed. Another consideration is to screen the woman alone, without the accompaniment of her partner, friends, family, or caregiver.[11] By creating an environment of nonjudgmental caring and concern, the health care provider can promote the trust that allows a patient to safely disclose violence and abuse.[11] Recognizing that disclosure may create a significant risk for the woman, building trust and providing a safe environment for disclosure should be the goal of the health care provider.[12]

INDICATORS OF ABUSE

During all interactions, health care providers should assess for indicators of abuse. These include injury-related, medical-related, and emotional indicators of abuse (**Boxes 1–3**).

Screening procedures for IPV, along with the awareness of abuse indicators, have the potential to significantly increase the identification of women who have been exposed to IPV. Identifications of IPV will enable the health care provider to offer the woman support, build trust, validate concerns, and offer community resources.[15]

NONLETHAL STRANGULATION

Strangulation is a serious indicator of IPV. Women are at least twice as likely as men to report having been strangled by an intimate partner.[16] There is an 800% increased risk of homicide for women who report strangulation in an abusive intimate relationship.[17] Even when there are few or subtle signs of strangulation, victims may still experience anoxia resulting in serious and permanent impairment or death.

Documentation includes statements by the victim in quotations, the use of any weapons, position of the assailant during the strangulation, and perceived duration of the strangulation. Injuries such as abrasions to the face or neck, or bruises on the arms may indicate defensive injuries. Petechiae above the level of the ligature, as well as scleral and subconjunctival hemorrhages, indicate an especially vigorous struggle. The loss of bowel and/or bladder control cannot be used to indicate the severity of the assault; however, it does indicate that a loss of consciousness has occurred. Evidence of neurologic impairment, unilateral weakness, loss of sensation, restlessness, and combativeness may be due to hypoxia. Some changes can be long-lasting and should be red flags for the provider when considering the potential of future lethal IPV.

Box 1
Injury-related indicators of abuse

1. Injury inconsistent with history provided

2. Injury related to motor vehicle accident

3. Multiple injuries in various stages of healing

4. Injuries covered up by clothing, make-up, or sunglasses

5. Patterned injuries, such as belt marks or implement imprint

6. Pregnancy injuries, especially to abdomen and chest

7. Injuries suggestive of defensive posture (inner aspect of forearms or top of head)

8. Common injuries that may indicate abuse: black eyes and injuries to teeth, neck, or head

Data from Refs.[4,12–14]

Box 2
Medical-related indicators of abuse

1. Somatic complaints (headache, gastrointestinal problems, stomach aches)

2. Evidence of strangulation

3. Acute psychiatric manifestations (suicide attempts)

4. Chronic psychiatric symptoms (anxiety, depression, posttraumatic stress disorder)

5. Chronic pain

6. Malnutrition, poor hygiene

Data from The Ohio domestic violence protocol for health care providers: standards of care. The Ohio Domestic Violence Network and the National Health Care Standards Campaign Committee Ohio. Chapter. 2012. Available at: https://www.odh.ohio.gov/-/media/ODH/ASSETS/Files/health/SADVP/DV_Protocol_122012.pdf?la=en. Accessed July 18, 2017; and Campbell J. Health consequences of intimate partner violence. Lancet 2002;359:1331–6.

Any individual who has been the victim of strangulation should be evaluated by an emergency provider who is familiar with the current standard of care. Recommendations for the medical-radiographic evaluation of acute adult nonfatal strangulation[18] have been released by the Training Institute on Strangulation Prevention, and should be readily accessible in every emergency department.

Conducting the Screening

There are many recommendations for conducting screenings for IPV (**Box 4**).

Provider Response to Screening

Findings from a negative screen with no indicators of abuse should be documented in the medical record and the health care provider should acknowledge concern for the safety and well-being of all women. If abuse arises in the future, information about resources can be provided. Document "Patient response negative to abuse screen," respect her response,[9,11] and offer educational material about IPV.[9,11]

When the woman has a negative screen but there are indicators that cause the health care provider to suspect abuse, acknowledge understanding and respect her response to the screen.[9] State your concerns directly to the woman and offer information that she may need in the future. Emphasize nonjudgmental support and willingness to help.[9,11] Address medical conditions and symptoms, and offer resources such as the National Domestic Violence hotline.[9]

Box 3
Emotional indicators of abuse

1. Fearfulness of partner

2. Hypervigilance of the woman and/or partner

3. Woman appears frightened, embarrassed, ashamed, or disoriented

4. Excessive distress about a minor injury, or little emotion apparent about a serious injury

5. Delay in seeking care

Data from Refs.[11,13,14]

Box 4
Recommendations for conducting the screening

Screening should

1. Be framed with an introductory sentence that establishes screening is a universal practice and not unique to the patient[11]
   - Example: "We've started talking to all of our women about safe and healthy relationships because it can have such a large impact on your health."[11]
   - Example: "I don't know if this is a problem for you but many of my female patients are dealing with abusive relationships. Some are too afraid or uncomfortable to bring it up themselves, so I've started asking about it routinely."[19]

2. Discuss confidentiality with her and disclose state mandated laws[11]
   - Example: "Before we get started, I want you to know that everything here is confidential, meaning that I won't talk to anyone else about what is said unless you tell me that...(insert the laws in your state about what is necessary to disclose)."[11]

3. Use questions that are direct, specific, and easy to understand
   - Example: "Has your partner ever hit, choked, or physically hurt you?" (Hurt includes being hit, slapped, kicked, bitten, pushed, or shoved.)[11]

4. Use gender-neutral terms, such as "your partner" instead of "your boyfriend"

5. Be presented in the woman's primary language and be culturally appropriate (If an interpreter is needed locate a professional interpreter, do not use a family member or friend.)[11]

Data from Intimate partner violence. Committee opinion No. 518. American College of Obstetricians and Gynecologists. Obstet Gynecol 2012;119:412–7; and Stanford Medicine. Domestic abuse. Stanford University; 2017. Available at: http://domesticabuse.stanford.edu/screening/how.html. Accessed July 16, 2017.

When the screen is positive for abuse, write "positive screen for abuse." Acknowledge that there is a concern for her safety, address the trauma, and develop a safety plan (**Box 5**).[9,11]

DOCUMENTATION

In a study by Gerber and colleagues,[20] results indicated that medical record documentation for IPV was insufficient and failed to completely document the encounter. To effectively address the safety, medical, and legal needs of women who present with suspected or confirmed exposure to IPV, health care providers must do a better job. Complete documentation can assist the efforts of the legal system to address the violence and abuse.

For health care providers, documentation is among the most effective tools for recording an encounter. In situations in which IPV is suspected or confirmed, the health care provider's accurate and objective documentation of the event is vital to the continuity of care, justification for specific clinical recommendations, and legal evidence collection. Ensuring that documentation of IPV is complete and accurate has the potential to objectively serve as useable evidence for legal proceedings and assists with consistency of care from visit to visit and among health care providers.[20,21] Medical documentation can be submitted to the courts for the purpose of obtaining orders of protection. In addition, accurate documentation can support a woman's report of abuse and reinforce reports generated by law enforcement[21] (**Box 6**).

Box 5
Recommendations for positive screen for abuse

1. Thank her for having enough trust to disclose the abuse.
   - Example: "Thank you for telling me. I am concerned for your safety."

2. Acknowledge it is not her fault.
   - Example: "It is not your fault. There is help available."

3. Assess for immediate danger, assist with development of a safety plan, or consult with specialists who can provide this service.

4. Offer community resources and referrals for safety, education, caretaking, and support services. Remember that a local advocacy agency for domestic violence is among the most reliable resources.

5. Provide her with the national and/or local domestic violence hotline telephone number and other educational materials related to IPV.

6. Assist her with the processes for informing law enforcement, if the woman is agreeable, or when mandated by state law.

7. Document the abuse, health effects, or injuries relevant to her care using recognized forensic guidelines.

8. Maintain appropriate clinical follow-up.

9. Consider making a report to child protective services if children are involved and when required by state law.

Data from Liebschutz J, Rothman E. Intimate-partner violence–what physicians can do. N Engl J Med 2012;367(22):2071–3; and Intimate partner violence. The American College of Obstetricians and Gynecologists. 2012. Available at: https://www.acog.org/Resources-And-Publications/Committee-Opinions/Committee-on-Health-Care-for-Underserved-Women/Intimate-Partner-Violence. Accessed July 16, 2017.

Box 6
Recommendations for medical documentation

1. Photographs of injuries related to IPV

2. A body map to further identify the location of injuries

3. Documentation that is clearly written and legible

4. Document history of the abuse and description of how injuries were received using the woman's own words (in quotation marks)

5. Avoid using judgmental words such as "alleges" and "patient claims"

6. Use phrases such as "patient reports" or "patient states"

7. Record her demeanor

8. Document her perception of safety and risk

Data from The Ohio domestic violence protocol for health care providers: standards of care. The Ohio Domestic Violence Network and the National Health Care Standards Campaign Committee Ohio. Chapter. 2012. Available at: https://www.odh.ohio.gov/-/media/ODH/ASSETS/Files/health/SADVP/DV_Protocol_122012.pdf?la=en. Accessed July 18, 2017; and Isaac N, Enos P. Documenting domestic violence: how health care providers can help victims. National Institute of Justice Web site. 2001. Available at: https://www.ncjrs.gov/pdffiles1/nij/188564.pdf. Accessed July 20, 2017.

If a woman does not disclose abuse, document that she did not disclose abuse and document any concerns that support suspected exposure to abuse. In addition, document any resources provided.

Resources

The role of the health care provider is to identify and document abuse while remaining nonjudgmental and sensitive to the woman, to document findings and care provided in the medical record, and to offer information, resources, and referrals. There is a significant health benefit to ensuring women have access to resources.[22] Insufficient or lack of access to resources can have adverse health consequences, which include emotional, social, and physical effects.[23]

There are several barriers to consider when offering access to resources. First, a woman may not perceive the abuse to be serious enough to require access to community resources.[23] Second, if a woman is not provided information inclusive of all the resources offered, she may not be aware of resources that may best fit her needs.[23] Third, the abuser may assert control that prohibits her from safely accessing resources.[23] Resources exist within most health care agencies for social workers to connect women to specialized assistance and referrals. Community-based advocates also play an important role in effective assistance, allowing the health care provider to manage the health issues related to the abuse. The woman is the best person to know how to stay safe during an emergency (**Box 7**).

Other resources used by women who have been exposed to IPV include[23] mental health resources (counseling, support groups, inpatient programs), social service agencies (shelters, food banks), medical and legal resources, and services offered through faith-based organizations.

When the health care provider focuses on the woman leaving an abusive relationship or situation, a sense of frustration may develop if she chooses to stay. The decision to leave and the first 6 months after leaving are the most dangerous times in an abusive relationship. Providers who do not recognize the enormous difficulty in the woman leaving home may label her as noncompliant and blame her for continuing the abuse. Eventually, this attitude becomes apparent to the woman and may result in her backing away from disclosure or acting on the providers' recommendations. The goal of the interaction with the woman is not for her to leave the relationship. The goal is to increase the safety of the woman and her family. Leaving an abusive relationship is a process that often requires months or years of planning, and may involve multiple attempts of leaving and returning.

Box 7
Recommendations for assisting intimate partner violence victims

- Discuss who to call during a crisis
- Encourage planning an escape route and a place to go in a crisis
- Identify the important documents the woman needs to have readily available (ie, birth certificates, Social Security cards, marriage and driver's license, school records, credit cards)
- Recommend having clothing, keys, medications, telephone numbers, and money readily available in a secure location

SAFETY PLANNING

Safety planning is an important part of the process when considering the needs of a woman who has experienced IPV and health care providers should be informed about the components of safety planning. The woman must be an active participant in her safety plan because she is the best judge of her own safety needs. The health care provider will need to recognize that the safety plan may not just address the needs of a woman who is leaving the abuser but may also include a safety plan for staying with the abuser. The best safety plan is a plan that has been tailored to her safety needs and addresses recommendations put forth by the Domestic Violence Resource Center.[24]

Explosive incidents can put women at great risk for injury. Factors to when planning for a woman's safety during an explosive incident are listed in **Box 8**.

In some cases the abuser is removed from the home and the woman opts to stay in the home. When this scenario occurs, consider advising the woman to secure a restraining order of protection, inform neighbors to alert law enforcement if the abuser is seen in the neighborhood or near the property, change all door locks, reinforce windows for additional security, and change pass codes and/or alarm codes.[24]

When a woman decides to leave, safety planning is essential due to the danger associated with her leaving. Working closely with her, safety planning should include consideration of the factors listed in **Box 9**.

Restraining orders or orders of protection are usually part of the process and are designed to protect the woman from the abuser. When developing a safety plan, if a restraining order or order of protection is in place, be sure to consider the factors listed in **Box 10**.

Priority should be given to safety when working with women who have been exposed to IPV. Collaborating with her is the most effective approach to developing a safety plan. Consideration of her situation is of the utmost importance when working to ensure that she is protected.

LEGAL AND CONFIDENTIALITY CONSIDERATIONS

Mandatory reporting laws vary from state to state, and it is crucial for health care providers to know and understand the mandatory laws in their state and how those laws affect health care providers responding to victims of IPV. Reporting child abuse is

---

Box 8
Recommendations for safety planning during explosive incidents

1. Plan for how to exit the home from different rooms in the house. If an argument is in progress, consider staying out of the kitchen where there are potential weapons, such as knives; or bathrooms, where the space is limited and there is a potential for increased injuries related to falls.

2. During an explosive event, find a room with a lock.

3. Document the abuse and take pictures of injuries.

4. Create a code word that will alert family, friends, and neighbors to contact law enforcement.

5. Have a plan for where to go if leaving is imminent and consider having clothes at that site for yourself and children, if applicable.

6. Instruct children not to get involved in the argument, despite a desire to help.

Box 9
Recommendations for the woman for safety planning when she decides to leave

1. Open bank accounts or set up credit cards in your name only
2. Change telephone number and block caller identification
3. Create new email account, change all passwords and personal identification (PIN) numbers
4. Leave important documents, money, keys, and clothes with a trusted person
5. Identify people you can stay with or who can lend money
6. Keep national and local hotline numbers available
7. Keep the number of community agencies available
8. Review, revise, and rehearse safety plan as needed
9. If children are involved, notify the school about any changes and advise them not to disclose address information
10. Inform employer of situation; to prevent access to you during work hours, provide a picture of the abuser
11. Change daily habits
12. Discuss safety plan with children related to times when they are not with you

Data from Domestic Violence Resource Center. Safety planning. Available at: http://www.dvrc-or.org/safety-planning/.

---

mandatory; however, reporting specific types of abuse related to victims 18 years of age and older who are competent may not be mandatory. Reporting is not required by law in many states. Mandatory laws were put in place to ensure the safety and security of individuals who experience abuse or certain injuries; however, with IPV the involvement of law enforcement could put the woman at increased risk for serious harm.[11] As a health care provider it is important to discuss and disclose mandated reporting requirements and procedures, as well as the use of the woman's health information.[25] Mandatory reporting laws fall into 4 categories[25]:

1. States that require the reporting of injuries caused by weapons
2. States that mandate reporting for injuries caused in violation of criminal laws, as a result of violence, or through nonaccidental means
3. States that specifically address reporting in IPV cases
4. State that have no general mandatory reporting laws.

Box 10
Recommendations for the woman for safety planning when protection order is in place

- Keep restraining order or order of protection on you at all times
- Give a copy to a trusted friend or family member
- Inform family, friends, health care providers, employers, schools (if children are involved), and neighbors that you have a protective order
- Call law enforcement if abuser violates the order
- Consider alternate ways of staying safe until law enforcement arrives

Courtesy of Domestic Violence Resource Center, Washington County Oregon. Available at: http://www.dvrc-or.org/safety-planning/.

The individual autonomy of each woman must be balanced with the safety concern for making a report. By removing the legal mandate to report IPV to law enforcement, women are more willing to accept medical services and referrals.[25] A goal for health care providers when addressing the needs of women who have been exposed to IPV is to provide care that is ongoing and accessible.[25]

Check state laws for mandatory reporting requirements when children (in the absence of injury or risk of injury) witness IPV.[25] In cases when it is mandatory to report IPV (witnessed by child) the best approach for reporting includes the woman making the call to child protective services. This reduces the chances of her being charged with failure to protect, and can reinforce that the woman is providing a safe home environment.[9,25]

Health care providers must maintain confidentiality when caring for women who have experienced IPV. All policies, protocols, and practices related to the disclosure of private health information regarding IPV should respect a woman's autonomy and confidentiality, and should focus on the safety and health concerns of the woman.[12] A break in confidentiality may result in a greater risk to the woman. Hospitals and other health care organizations should consider policies that include health care providers discussing confidentiality and limits to confidentiality before assessing for IPV.[12,13] Disclosing the limits of confidentiality gives the decision-making power to the woman and allows her to decide what she is ready and willing to discuss with the health care provider.

SUMMARY

Health care providers must be knowledgeable about the processes for screening, documenting, and providing resources to women who have been exposed to or experienced IPV. Laws, policies, and standards of practice are constantly evolving but there are norms that should always be followed when working with these women. Those norms include listening, ensuring safety, promoting autonomy, coordinating services, and offering community resources. Building trust and implementing a victim-centered approach can significantly contribute to disclosure, which can lead to the victim becoming a survivor.

REFERENCES

1. Statistics. National Coalition against Domestic Violence Web Site. Available at: http://ncadv.org/learn-more/statistics. Accessed July 3, 2017.
2. Intimate partner violence: consequences. Centers for Disease Control and Prevention Web Site. 2017. Available at: https://www.cdc.gov/violenceprevention/intimatepartnerviolence/consequences.html. Accessed August 23, 2017.
3. Intimate partner violence: definitions. Centers for Disease Control and Prevention Web Site. 2017. Available at: https://www.cdc.gov/violenceprevention/intimate partnerviolence/definitions.html. Accessed August 23, 2017.
4. Foushee JP. Identifying domestic violence in patients. Radiol Technol 2016;88(2):218–21. Available at: http://www.radiologictechnology.org/content/88/2/218.extract.
5. Guerin B, de Oliveira Ortolan M. Analyzing domestic violence behaviors in their context: violence as a continuation of social strategies by other means. Behav Soc Issues 2017;26:5–26.
6. Nelson H, Bougatsos C, Blazina I. Screening women for intimate partner violence: a systematic review to update the 2004 U.S. Preventive Services Task Force Recommendation. Ann Intern Med 2012;156(1):796–808.

7. US Preventive Services Task Force. Draft update summary: intimate partner violence, elder abuse, and abuse of vulnerable 'adults: screening. U.S. Preventive Services Task Force; 2016. Available at: https://www.uspreventiveservicestaskforce.org/Page/Document/UpdateSummaryDraft/intimate-partner-violence-and-abuse-of-elderly-and-vulnerable-adults-screening1. Accessed September 15, 2017.

8. Health Resources and Services Administration (HRSA). Women's preventive health services: required health plan coverage guidelines. Rockville (MD): Health Resources and Services Administration, U.S. Department of Health and Human Services; 2012. Available(at: http://www.hrsa.gov/womensguidelines. Accessed July 3, 2017.

9. Liebschutz J, Rothman E. Intimate-partner violence–what physicians can do. N Engl J Med 2012;367(22):2071–3.

10. National Research Council. Confronting chronic neglect: the education and training of health professionals on family violence. Washington, DC: The National Academies Press; 2002.

11. Intimate partner violence. The American College of Obstetricians and Gynecologists. 2012. Available at: https://www.acog.org/Resources-And-Publications/Committee-Opinions/Committee-on-Health-Care-for-Underserved-Women/Intimate-Partner-Violence. Accessed July 16, 2017.

12. National consensus guidelines on identifying and responding to domestic violence victimization in healthcare settings. The Family Violence Prevention Fund. 2004. Available at: http://www.futureswithoutviolence.org/userfiles/file/Consensus.pdf. Accessed July 18, 2017.

13. The Ohio domestic violence protocol for health care providers: standards of care. The Ohio Domestic Violence Network and the National Health Care Standards Campaign Committee Ohio. Chapter. 2012. Available at: https://www.odh.ohio.gov/-/media/ODH/ASSETS/Files/health/SADVP/DV_Protocol_122012.pdf?la=en. Accessed July 18, 2017.

14. Campbell J. Health consequences of intimate partner violence. Lancet 2002;359: 1331–6.

15. Coker A, Smith P, McKeown R, et al. Frequency and correlates of intimate partner violence by type: physical, sexual, and psychological battering. Am J Public Health 2000;90:553–9.

16. Black MC, Basile KC, Breiding MJ. The National Intimate Partner and Sexual Violence Survey (NISVS). In: National Center for Injury Prevention and Control & C. f. D. C. a. Prevention. 2017. Available at: https://www.cdc.gov/violenceprevention/pdf/NISVS-StateReportBook.pdf. Accessed September 15, 2017.

17. Glass N, Laughon K, Campbell J, et al. Non-fatal strangulation is an important risk factor for homicide of women. J Emerg Med 2008;35(3):329–35.

18. Smock B, Sturgeon S. Recommendations for the medical/radiographic evaluation of acute adult, non-fatal strangulation. 2016. Available at: https://www.strangulationtraininginstitute.com/resources/library/medical-radiographic-imaging-recommendations. Accessed September 20, 2017.

19. Stanford Medicine. Domestic abuse. Stanford University; 2017. Available at: http://domesticabuse.stanford.edu/screening/how.html. Accessed July 16, 2017.

20. Gerber M, Leiter K, Hermann R, et al. How and why community hospital clinicians document a positive screen for intimate partner violence: a cross sectional study. BMC Fam Pract 2005;6(48):1–9.

21. Isaac N, Enos P. Documenting domestic violence: how health care providers can help victims. National Institute of Justice Web site. 2001. Available at: https://www.ncjrs.gov/pdffiles1/nij/188564.pdf. Accessed July 20, 2017.

22. Beeble M, Bybee D, Sullivan C. The impact of resource constraints on the psychological well-being of survivors of intimate partner violence over time. J Community Psychol 2010;38(8):943–59.

23. McLeod A, Hays D, Chang C. Female intimate partner violence survivors' experiences with accessing resources. J Couns Dev 2010;88:303–10.

24. Safety planning. Domestic Violence Resource Center Web site. 2014. Available at: http://www.dvrc-or.org/safety-planning/. Accessed September 3, 2017.

25. Mandatory reporting of domestic violence to law enforcement by health care providers: a guide for advocates working to respond to or amend reporting laws related to domestic violence. Date unavailable. Available at: https://www.futureswithoutviolence.org/userfiles/Mandatory_Reporting_of_DV_to_Law%20Enforcement_by_HCP.pdf. Accessed August 3, 2017.

Common Sexually Transmitted Infections in Women

Ashley L. Hodges, PhD, CRNP, WHNP-BC*,
Aimee Chism Holland, DNP, WHNP-BC, FNP-BC, RD

KEYWORDS

- Sexually transmitted infections • Vaginal infections • Women's health • Cervicitis
- Vaginal discharge

KEY POINTS

- The spread of sexually transmitted infections remains a significant public health issue in the United States.
- Screening women for infections of the vagina and cervix is essential because untreated infections may result in complications that have current and long-term health consequences and impact quality of life.
- The Centers for Disease Control and Prevention recently updated the Sexually Transmitted Diseases Treatment Guidelines in 2015 to provide the most current evidence-based guide for screening individuals across the lifespan for infections.

INTRODUCTION

The Centers for Disease Control and Prevention (CDC) updated the Sexually Transmitted Diseases Treatment Guidelines in 2015 to provide the most current evidence-based recommendations for screening and treating individuals across the lifespan. Prevalence rates among adolescents and young adults in the United States are highest among females for chlamydia, gonorrhea, and human papillomavirus (HPV).[1,2]

The spread of sexually transmitted infections (STIs) remains a significant health problem.[1] Approximately 20 million new STIs are diagnosed each year in the United States, of which almost half of them are identified in young people ages 15 to 24 year old.[2] In addition to age disparities, gender disparities also exist because women are diagnosed more frequently with STIs than men.[2] Both the age and gender

Disclosure Statement: The authors have no disclosures.
Department of Family, Community, and Health Systems, University of Alabama at Birmingham School of Nursing, 1701 University Boulevard, Birmingham, AL 35294-1210, USA
* Corresponding author.
E-mail address: ashleyhodges@uab.edu

disparities are of critical importance, because untreated STIs can lead to long-term health consequences for women, including infertility, ectopic pregnancy, chronic pelvic pain, cervical cancer, and chronic liver disease.[1,3]

Social, economic, and behavioral implications affecting the spread of STIs have been identified in the United States. The most important social factor impacting the spread of STIs in the United States is the stigma associated with discussing sex and STI screening.[4] Race and ethnicity factors associated with high rates of STIs include being African American, Hispanic, American Indian, or Alaskan Native.[2,3] Disadvantaged socioeconomic status populations and populations associated with high-risk behaviors are also at an increased risk of contracting an STI.[3]

National goals for reducing the spread of STIs and for increasing prevention of STIs are included in the Healthy People 2020 (HP2020) document. Health care providers play an important role in reducing STI rates by bridging knowledge gaps and removing access barriers. The Sexually Transmitted Diseases Treatment Guidelines document is an essential resource for meeting the HP2020 goals. This article summarizes critical information for health care providers to safely and effectively prevent and manage STIs for women across the lifespan.

BACTERIAL VAGINOSIS
Screening and Diagnosing

Screening for bacterial vaginosis (BV) is recommended for women presenting with vaginal discharge or odor. The diagnosis in the clinical setting is most often based on the Amsel criteria, which includes the presence of at least three of the following: grayish-white vaginal discharge, pH greater than 4.5, positive whiff test for a fishy odor in the presence of potassium hydroxide, or observation of clue cells under microscopy.[1] Researchers often use the Nugent criteria to diagnose BV using a gram-stained smear of discharge. Commercial diagnostic tests are also available for diagnosing BV.

Incidence/Prevalence

BV is the most common cause of discharge among women of reproductive age.[1] The most recent US National Health and Nutrition Examination Survey study noted the prevalence of BV at 29% among the general population in reproductive age women. The highest rates were reported among African American women followed by Mexican-American women and white women.[5] BV is predominantly diagnosed in sexually active women.

Risk Factors

Sexual activity, douching, and a lack of lactobacillus in the vagina are common risk factors for BV. A diagnosis of BV increases the risks for acquisition of other STIs, including human immunodeficiency virus (HIV), gonorrhea, chlamydia, and herpes simplex virus (HSV).[1] Therefore, women diagnosed with BV should be screened for STIs.

Treatment

Treatment is recommended in symptomatic women. In addition to the treatments listed in **Box 1**, recent studies have provided promising outcomes with the addition of lactic acid vaginal gel and probiotics, such as *Lactobacillus reuteri* and *Lactobacillus rhamnosus*, in the treatment of recurrent BV.[6–8]

> **Box 1**
> **BV treatment**
>
> *Primary regimens*
>
> 1. Metronidazole 500 mg orally twice daily for 7 days (except first trimester of pregnancy)[a]
>
> 2. Metronidazole gel 0.75% (5 g) vaginally for 5 nights[a]
>
> 3. Clindamycin cream 2% (5 g) vaginally for 7 nights
>
> *Alternative treatments choices*
>
> 1. Tinidazole 2 g orally once daily for 2 days
>
> 2. Tinidazole 1 g orally once daily for 5 days
>
> 3. Clindamycin 300 mg orally twice daily for 7 days
>
> 4. Clindamycin ovules 100 mg vaginally for 3 nights
>
> [a] Caution patient not to use alcohol during and for 24 to 48 hours after dosing.

Prevention/Vaccination

Limiting the number of sex partners and avoiding douching is protective against BV. Abstinence is the only reliable preventive measure identified. Additional studies are needed to support the use of lactic acid products and probiotics to prevent BV.

Special Populations

Symptomatic BV diagnosed during pregnancy increases the risk of premature rupture of membranes, preterm labor, preterm birth, intra-amniotic infection, and postpartum endometritis. Therefore, treatment is recommended for all symptomatic women during pregnancy.[1] After the first trimester, oral metronidazole may be used during pregnancy to treat BV because it poses low fetal risks.[1]

DESQUAMATIVE INFLAMMATORY VAGINITIS
Screening and Diagnosing

There is no specific screening test for desquamative inflammatory vaginitis (DIV). Screening is only recommended when common vaginal infections are excluded in women presenting with a chronic purulent discharge, vestibule-vaginal irritation, or dyspareunia. In addition to wet mount and pH evaluations, a thorough history and inspection of the vagina should be performed. Common characteristics of DIV observed with a wet prep examination include a lack of lactobacillus, an increased number of parabasal epithelial cells, and an increased number of white blood cells.[9] A test measuring pH should be used to confirm a base environment greater than four.[9] DIV is not considered an STI, but rather a chronic inflammatory syndrome of unknown cause.

Incidence/Prevalence

The incidence of women diagnosed with DIV is between 0.8% and 4.3% as reflected in studies performed in vulvovaginal clinics.[9] However, research has yet to suggest the prevalence of DIV. DIV occurs in premenopausal, perimenopausal, and postmenopausal women and is diagnosed predominantly in perimenopausal women of white decent.[10]

Risk Factors

Known risk factors for DIV include sexual activity, white race, and perimenopausal status. The cause is unknown, but researchers believe this is caused by an alteration in vaginal flora and pH balance.

Treatment

This non-STI vaginal syndrome may require treatment more than one time (**Box 2**).

Prevention/Vaccination

Limited research is available regarding the prevention of DIV. However, a correlation exists between a healthy vaginal environment and a pH between 3.8 and 4.5.

TRICHOMONIASIS
Screening and Diagnosing

Trichomoniasis is a genitourinary infection with the protozoan *Trichomonas vaginalis*. Most persons infected with trichomoniasis (70%–85%) have minimal to no symptoms, allowing the infection to go untreated for months to years.[1] Screening should be considered for women receiving care in high-prevalence settings and in women considered at high risk for STIs. Diagnostic testing should be performed on women presenting for evaluation of vaginal discharge. Symptomatic women generally present with a purulent, malodorous, thin discharge with or without vulvar irritation. Some women may complain of burning, pruritus, dysuria, frequency, lower abdominal pain, or dyspareunia during the acute phase. With chronic infection, vaginal discharge may be minimal, and the woman may present with or without pruritus and dyspareunia.[11] Postcoital bleeding may also occur.

The most common method for diagnosing trichomoniasis is wet-mount microscopy of vaginal secretions. However, the low sensitivity of this method at 51% to 65% declines rapidly if evaluation is delayed beyond 1 hour after collection.[12] On wet mount, the presence of motile, jerking, and spinning trichomonads is diagnostic. Nucleic acid amplification testing (NAAT) is the recommended diagnostic method and is conducted on vaginal, endocervical, or urine specimens. In addition, cultures can be performed on vaginal secretions or urine; however, urine culture is less sensitive. There are also rapid diagnostic kits and positive rapid antigen or nucleic acid probe tests available. Although there may be an incidental finding on Pap test, it is not considered a reliable diagnostic method for trichomoniasis. However, specificity is high in positive results and therefore should be treated.[11,12]

Box 2
DIV treatment

Initial treatment[9,10]

Clindamycin 2% (5 g) vaginally each night for 3 weeks; maintenance dose twice weekly for 2 months

Relapse treatment choices

1. Compounded 10% hydrocortisone (5 g) cream vaginally each night for 3 weeks; maintenance dose twice weekly for 2 months
2. In mild cases 25 mg hydrocortisone suppository vaginally twice daily for 3 weeks; maintenance dose 25 mg three times weekly for 2 months

Rectal and oral screening are not recommended because of lack of evidence for rectal or oral infections. Routine screening at the first prenatal visit during pregnancy is only recommended if the woman is HIV-positive. The CDC recommends routine annual screening for all women infected with HIV.[1]

Retesting in women positive for trichomoniasis is recommend for all sexually active women within 3 months following treatment because of the high reinfection rate. NAAT can be performed 2 weeks after completing treatment, but providers should retest again at the 3-month mark.[1]

Incidence/Prevalence

Trichomoniasis is the most prevalent non-viral STI in the United States, with an estimated 3.7 million cases.[1] The actual prevalence is difficult to identify because of several factors: trichomoniasis is not a reportable STI, number of asymptomatic/undiagnosed cases, and low sensitivity of the most commonly used diagnostic method (wet mount microscopy). Significant disparities exist in race with 13% of black women affected compared with 1.7% of white non-Hispanic women.[1]

Risk Factors

Trichomoniasis is sexually transmitted most often between male and female, and female-to-female. Coinfection rates with BV are high at 60% to 80%.[13] Women who are HIV-positive are at greater risk of contracting trichomoniasis.

Treatment

All women diagnosed with trichomoniasis should be treated, whether symptomatic or asymptomatic. Patients should be treated with 5-nitroimidazole drugs (metronidazole or tinidazole) as a single 2-g oral dose. If not tolerated, an alternate is metronidazole, 500 mg orally twice a day for 7 days. No alcohol should be consumed during and for 24 hours after metronidazole treatment and for 72 hours after tinidazole treatment.[1] Patients with known 5-nitroimidazole allergies should be referred for desensitization. During treatment, the patient and all partners should abstain from sex until treatment is completed.[11]

Prevention/Vaccination

There is no vaccine for the prevention of trichomoniasis. Consistent condom use and limiting the number of sexual partners can reduce the risk of transmission. If left untreated, trichomoniasis may result in urethritis or cystitis. Trichomoniasis has also been associated with cervical neoplasia, post-hysterectomy cuff cellulitis or abscess, and infertility.[1]

Special Populations

Adverse outcomes of trichomoniasis in pregnancy are possible. These include premature rupture of the membranes, preterm delivery, and delivery of a low-birth-weight infant. Treatment in pregnancy is the same as treatment in the nonpregnant woman.[11]

HUMAN PAPILLOMAVIRUS
Screening and Diagnosing

Initiation of routine screening for high-risk, oncogenic types of HPV is recommended in women at age 30 years as a cotest with cervical cytology to screen for cervical cancer and should be repeated every 5 years.[1] Primary screening for high-risk HPV types 16 and 18 with reflex cytology is considered an alternative option for cervical cancer screening and may be initiated at age 25 years. This should be repeated no sooner than every 3 years until the 65 years of age.[14] Routine screening for nononcogenic types of HPV associated with genital warts and oral lesions is not recommended.[1]

Incidence/Prevalence

HPV is considered the most common STI in the United States with an estimated prevalence of 20 million infections and annual incidence estimated at 5.5 million infections.[15] HPV presentation varies from genital, oropharyngeal, and anal warts to vulvar, vaginal, cervical, oropharyngeal, and anal cancer. HPV incidence is similar between African American and white women, but African American women have higher rates of high-risk, persistent HPV types documented.[15] Highest HPV infection rates are among adolescents and young adult females following sexual debut.[2]

Risk Factors

The primary factor influencing HPV infection among women is sexual activity, specifically early debut and the number of lifetime sex partners.[15] Other risk factors include absence of condom use, history of an STI, race, immunodeficiency, cigarette smoking, and circumcision status of partner.[15] Research confirms that HPV is contracted from contact with a skin surface where the virus is located to another skin surface, supporting why barrier method use is important for sexually active women. However, it is important to mention that women who have never been sexually active and children have also been diagnosed with HPV, supporting the knowledge that the virus can spread by hand to genital contact.[15]

Treatment

There is no cure for this virus; however, most HPV infections, including genital warts, cervical infections, and vulvar infections, routinely do not require treatment because they resolve within 6 to 12 months of onset.[15] Even though genital warts are self-limiting women often seek treatment options because of aesthetic reasons. Treatment options are listed in **Box 3**.

Persistent high-risk HPV infections that do not resolve are observed with cytology and HPV screening. Histologic procedural options approved to evaluate and treat cervical HPV infections include colposcopy-guided biopsies and diagnostic excisional procedures. The four approved excisional procedures routinely performed to remove cervical intraepithelial neoplasia include (1) laser conization, (2) cold-knife conization, (3) loop electrosurgical excision procedure, and (4) loop electrosurgical conization.

A vulvar biopsy is used to identify HPV infection–related vulvar intraepithelial neoplasia. Treatment options for vulvar intraepithelial neoplasia include wide local excision, partial or total skinning of the vulva, ablative therapy, and topical treatment. Surgical excision is the primary treatment option performed for vulvar intraepithelial neoplasia.

Prevention/Vaccination

Primary prevention of HPV with vaccination is approved for females between the ages of 9 and 26 years old. An annual well-woman examination is helpful for identifying problems caused by HPV. Routine and accurate use of latex condoms may also reduce the risk of contracting HPV. Smoking cessation, healthy habits supporting a healthy immune system, and limiting the number of sex partners are suggested for lowering HPV infection risks.

Box 3
HPV treatment

Topical options

1. Podofilox

2. Trichloroacetic acid

3. Bichloroacetic acid

4. 5-Fluorouracil

5. Sinecatechins

6. Imiquimod

Surgical options

1. Cryoablation

2. Laser ablation

3. Electrocautery

4. Ultrasonic aspiration

5. Excision

Data from Palefsky JM. Human papillomavirus infections: epidemiology and disease associations. Available at: https://www.uptodate.com/contents/human-papillomavirus-infections-epidemiology-and-disease-associations?search=human-papillomavirus-uinfections-epidemiology-and-disease-associations&source=search_result&selectedTitle=1~150&usage_type=default&display_rank=1. Accessed March 13, 2018.

Special Populations

An elevation in hormone levels and the decrease in cell-mediated immunity are thought to be the rationale for genital warts proliferation during pregnancy. Most available treatments are contraindicated during pregnancy; therefore, fetal well-being should be considered when selecting an option. Topical trichloroacetic acid is the preferred treatment option for genital warts during pregnancy, followed by cryoablation, because neither option causes harmful fetal effects. Vertical transmission in the form of juvenile-onset respiratory papillomatosis is rare, but remains a risk when women are diagnosed with HPV during pregnancy. Studies have investigated the use of elective cesarean delivery and condyloma treatment as protective options; however, neither provided benefits against fetal transmission.[16,17] Cesarean delivery is indicated if vaginal or vulvar warts obstruct the birth canal.[17]

HERPES SIMPLEX VIRUS
Screening and Diagnosing

Routine screening for HSV-1 or HSV-2 is not recommended in asymptomatic adolescents and adults.[18] Depending on clinical presentation, HSV may be diagnosed by viral culture, polymerase chain reaction, direct fluorescence antibody, and type-specific serologic tests. When active lesions are present cell culture and polymerase chain reaction–based testing are preferred. Polymerase chain reaction–based testing has the greatest overall sensitivity and specificity.[1,18]

A positive serology indicates present or past infection. However, further diagnostic evaluation of an active genital ulcer is needed in the case of a positive HSV IgG antibody serology. There are many causes for genital ulcers; therefore, the IgG antibody cannot be used alone for diagnosis. If there is an HSV-positive culture in an

HSV-seronegative patient, the result is considered strong evidence of primary infection.[18] Serologic tests for HSV-1 cannot differentiate between oral and anogential infection, whereas positive serology for HSV-2 indicates an anogenital infection.

Incidence/Prevalence

There are two types of HSV that cause genital herpes: HSV-1 and HSV-2. Approximately 50 million persons in the United States are infected with HSV-2, the most common cause.[1] Despite this, there has been an increase in the number of HSV-1 cases of genital herpes infection. Most cases of HSV are subclinical and go undiagnosed.[19]

Risk Factors

The seroprevalence of HSV increases with age and number of sexual partners. It is more common among women than men.[18]

Treatment

There is no cure for this viral infection. During the primary outbreak, providers have multiple treatment options to consider in meeting the needs of the patient. Antiviral therapy for recurrent HSV is taken episodically during recurrent outbreaks or as suppressive therapy. Patients often choose suppressive therapy, which decreases the risk of transmission to sexual partners. These options for treatment are provided in **Box 4.**[1]

Box 4
HSV treatment (all options are oral)

Primary outbreak options
1. Acyclovir, 200 mg 5 times a day for 7 to 10 days
2. Acyclovir, 400 mg 3 times a day for 7 to 10 days
3. Valacyclovir, 1 g twice a day for 7 to 10 days
4. Famciclovir, 250 mg 3 times a day for 7 to 10 days

Episodic treatment options
1. Acyclovir, 400 mg 3 times a day for 5 days
2. Acyclovir, 800 mg twice a day for 5 days
3. Acyclovir, 800 mg three times a day for 2 days
4. Valacyclovir, 500 mg twice a day for 3 days
5. Valacyclovir, 1 g once a day for 5 days
6. Famciclovir, 125 mg twice a day for 5 days
7. Famciclovir, 250 mg; 500 mg to start, then 250 mg twice a day for 2 days
8. Famciclovir, 1 g twice daily for 1 day

Suppressive therapy options
1. Acyclovir, 400 mg twice a day
2. Valacyclovir, 500 mg once daily
3. Valacyclovir, 1 g once a day for patients with more than 10 episodes/year
4. Famciclovir, 250 mg twice daily

Data from Workowski KA, Bolan GA, Centers for Disease Control and Prevention. Sexually transmitted diseases treatment guidelines, 2015. MMWR Recomm Rep 2015;64(RR-03):1–137.

Patients with severe disease during the primary outbreak may develop central nervous system complications (aseptic meningitis, encephalitis, or transverse myelitis), end-organ disease including hepatitis or pneumonitis, and disseminated HSV. In these cases, patients require hospitalization.[1]

Prevention/Vaccination

Although studies are underway, there is no vaccine for prevention of HSV. Consistent condom use and limiting the number of sexual partners can reduce the risk of transmission. Avoiding exposure during a partner's active outbreak has shown some benefit; however, vital shedding occurs even in the absence of active lesions. Transmission of the HSV virus to the discordant partner is reduced though suppressive therapy in the infected individual.[1]

Special Populations

Immunocompromised patients with HIV may have prolonged or severe episodes of genital, oral, or perianal herpes. The initiation of antiretroviral therapy may reduce the severity and frequency of HSV-associated genital lesions. Clinical manifestations may worsen during immune reconstitution early after initiation of antiretroviral therapy. Suppressive or episodic therapy at higher doses can decrease the clinical manifestations of HSV among persons with HIV infection.[1]

During pregnancy, the major concern relates to the morbidity and mortality associated with neonatal HSV infection.[1] Most often, the woman has a newly acquired subclinical HSV infection and vertical transmission to the newborn occurs during delivery. When women contract HSV late in pregnancy, a maternal-fetal medicine specialist should be consulted. At the time of delivery, women without any prodromal or active symptoms or herpetic lesions may be delivered vaginally. However, if there is any indication of an outbreak, cesarean delivery is indicated.[1] Suppressive therapy starting after 36 weeks' gestation has been shown to decrease the frequency of recurrence at delivery.[20]

MYCOPLASMA GENITALIUM
Screening and Diagnosing

Mycoplasma genitalium (MG) is the most recent STI included in the CDC STD treatment guidelines; however, this infection was initially described in the literature in 1981.[21] It is difficult to culture this organism because of the slow replication cycle; therefore, NAAT with a vaginal swab is recommended.[22] Common symptoms observed in women include vaginal discharge and cervicitis; however, in some cases there are no symptoms.[1] MG has been isolated in cases of pelvic inflammatory disease. Therefore, screening should be considered for women presenting with clinical cervicitis.

Incidence/Prevalence

MG is not as prevalent in the United States as in other countries. Less than 1% of women in the general population have received the diagnosis.[23] However, there is a higher prevalence, up to 38%, among of STI clinic patients.[24] Globally, the prevalence in women is between 1% and 6.4%.[25]

Risk Factors

Young age, tobacco use, nonwhite race, frequent sexual activity, and a high number of sex partners are common risk factors for contracting MG. Coinfections with MG and other STIs have been reported. Chlamydia has the highest documented coinfection rate.[23]

Treatment

One gram of azithromycin orally is the preferred treatment of MG followed by a 7-day oral regimen of 100 mg doxycycline twice daily. Resistance to both antibiotics is 50%.[1] A 400-mg dose of moxifloxacin for 10 to 14 days should be reserved for treatment when azithromycin and doxycycline are not effective cures, because no resistance has been documented. Partner treatment is important.

Prevention/Vaccination

Routine condom use should be encouraged to help prevent the spread of MG. A test of cure is not recommended after treatment if the patient is asymptomatic.

Special Populations

No recommendations have been published regarding screening and treating for MG during pregnancy. However, evidence suggests that MG may be associated with preterm birth and miscarriages.[26]

CHLAMYDIA
Screening and Diagnosing

The CDC recommends annual screening for all women younger than 25 years old because asymptomatic infection is common. Complications from untreated infection include pelvic inflammatory disease, infertility, ectopic pregnancy, and chronic pelvic pain. Annual screening is recommended for women 25 years and older who have increased risks for infection.[1] Screening during pregnancy is recommended for all women at the first prenatal appointment and again during the third trimester for women younger than 25 years old and/or at increased risk for infection.[1]

Confirm urogenital diagnosis in women by screening urine or swabbing the endocervical canal or vagina. Vaginal or endocervical swabs are more sensitive than testing urine and can be self-collected by the patient or obtained by the provider.[1] Other anatomic sites that may require screening based on sexual practices and exposure include the urethra, anus, and oropharynx. The gold standard for screening is the NAAT, followed by a culture.

A test of cure is not recommended after treatment unless symptoms persist, reinfection is suspected, or treatment adherence is a concern. If warranted, providers should wait until 3 to 4 weeks following treatment to perform a test of cure.[1]

Incidence/Prevalence

Chlamydia is the most frequently reported infection in the United States.[1] In 2015, the incidence rate was 478.8 cases per 100,000 individuals.[1] Prevalence is highest among women younger than 25 years old. The highest rates in the United States have been documented in African American women.[1] Chlamydia infection is common among heterosexual, homosexual, and bisexual women.[2]

Risk Factors

Age less than 25 years, new sex partner, inconsistent use of condoms, and history of previous chlamydia infection are common risk factors identified with contracting the infection. Race, socioeconomic status, and history of STIs are other risk factors to consider.

Treatment

Prompt treatment (**Box 5**) should be provided to avoid complications associated with chlamydia. Safe treatment options during pregnancy vary, with the primary recommended regimen being a single 1-g oral dose of azithromycin. Alternative regimens include 500 mg of amoxicillin orally three times daily for 7 days, or various options of erythromycin.[1]

Prevention/Vaccination

Patient-centered counseling focused on prevention of chlamydia is considered an important responsibility of providers. Routine use of condoms should be encouraged as an effective option for the prevention of chlamydia.[1] Teaching patients diagnosed with chlamydia about the importance of referring sex partners for evaluation and treatment, along with the importance of abstinence until partner treatment is obtained can help prevent future infections.

Special Populations

Screening and treating for chlamydia during pregnancy is vital for the newborn. Chlamydia can cause ophthalmia neonatorum and chlamydia pneumonia among neonates delivered vaginally. It can also lead to premature rupture of membranes and preterm delivery if left untreated.

GONORRHEA
Screening and Diagnosing

Screening guidelines recommended by the CDC for gonorrhea and chlamydia are the same because both are often diagnosed as coinfections. Complications from untreated gonorrhea are the same as those listed for chlamydia. Cervical discharge and postcoital bleeding may or may not be present with a gonorrhea infection.

Incidence/Prevalence

Gonorrhea is the second most commonly reported infection in the United States.[2] In 2015, the incidence rate was 123.9 cases per 100,000 individuals.[1] Prevalence is highest among women younger than 25 years old. As with chlamydia, the highest rates are documented among African American women.[1]

Box 5
Chlamydia

Recommended options

1. Azithromycin 1 g orally, one time

2. Doxycycline 100 mg orally twice daily for 7 days[a]

Alternative options

1. Erythromycin base 500 mg orally four times daily for 7 days

2. Levofloxacin 500 mg orally daily for 7 days[b]

3. Ofloxacin 300 mg orally twice daily for 7 days[b]

[a] Doxycycline is contraindicated in the second and third trimesters of pregnancy.
[b] Use alternative drugs during pregnancy.
Data from Workowski KA, Bolan GA, Centers for Disease Control and Prevention. Sexually transmitted diseases treatment guidelines, 2015. MMWR Recomm Rep 2015;64(RR-03):1–137.

Box 6
Gonorrhea

Dual-therapy regimen

Ceftriaxone 250 mg intramuscularly, plus 1 g oral dose of azithromycin (once)

Alternative treatment

Cefixime 400 mg orally, plus 1 g oral dose of azithromycin (once)

Risk Factors

Risk factors for gonorrhea and chlamydia are the same. Refer to the previous section for a list of risk factors associated with both infections.

Treatment

Prompt treatment is recommended to avoid complications. Antibiotic treatment resistance is an important issue. As a result, the CDC updated the recommended treatment regimen to reflect a following dual-therapy regimen (**Box 6**).[1]

Prevention/Vaccination

Using condoms and other barrier methods, limiting the number of sex partners, and practicing abstinence should be encouraged as preventative measures for contracting gonorrhea. Partner treatment is also important for preventing reinfection.

Special Populations

Untreated maternal gonorrhea infections, present at the time of delivery, may result in neonatal ophthalmia neonatorum or neonatal gonococcal arthritis. Neonatal ophthalmia neonatorum may result in blindness if not treated. Neonatal gonococcal arthritis often results in children resisting to move their limbs secondary to pain.

The recommended treatment regimen for gonorrhea during pregnancy is the same option for nonpregnant women. Screening during the third trimester is essential to help prevent maternal and neonatal complications.

SUMMARY: IMPLICATIONS FOR PRACTICE

Health care providers play an essential role in preventing complications from and reducing the spread of STIs in the United States. By bridging knowledge gaps and removing access barriers, health care providers can help meet the HP2020 goals to decrease the spread of STIs. Health care providers are encouraged to use the Sexually Transmitted Diseases Treatment Guidelines, 2015 document for providing safe and effective care.

REFERENCES

1. Workowski KA, Bolan GA, Centers for Disease Control and Prevention. Sexually transmitted diseases treatment guidelines, 2015. MMWR Recomm Rep 2015; 64(RR-03):1–137.
2. Centers for Disease Control and Prevention. Sexually transmitted disease surveillance, 2015. Available at: https://www.cdc.gov/std/stats/. Accessed March 13, 2018.
3. Office of Disease Prevention and Health Promotion. 2017. Available at: https://www.healthypeople.gov/2020/topics-objectives/topic/sexually-transmitted-diseases/objectives. Accessed March 13, 2018.

4. Shepherd L, Harwood H. The role of STI-related attitudes on screening attendance in young adults. Psychol Health Med 2017;22(6):753–8.
5. CDC. Bacterial vaginosis is the most common vaginal infection in women ages 15-44. 2017. Available at: https://www.cdc.gov/std/bv/stats.htm. Accessed March 13, 2018.
6. Sobel J. Bacterial vaginosis: treatment. 2017. Available at: www.uptodate.com/contents/bacterial-vaginosis-treatment. Accessed March 13, 2018.
7. Happel AU, Jaumdaly SZ, Pidwell T, et al. Probiotics for vaginal health in South Africa: what is on retailers' shelves? BMC Womens Health 2017;17(1):7.
8. Tachedjian G, Aldunate M, Bradshaw CS, et al. The role of lactic acid production by probiotic *Lactobacillus* species in vaginal health. Res Microbiol 2017. https://doi.org/10.1016/j.resmic.2017.04.001.
9. Reichman O, Sobel J. Desquamative inflammatory vaginitis. Best Pract Res Clin Obstet Gynaecol 2014;28(7):1042–50.
10. Sobel J. Desquamative inflammatory vaginitis. 2017. Available at: www.uptodate.com/contents/desquamative-inflammatory-vaginitis. Accessed March 13, 2018.
11. Sobel J. Trichomoniasis. 2017. Available at: https://www.uptodate.com/contents/trichomoniasis. Accessed March 13, 2018.
12. Stoner KA, Rabe LK, Meyn LA, et al. Survival of trichomonas vaginalis in wet preparation and on wet mount. Sex Transm Infect 2013;89:485–8.
13. Sobel JD, Subramanian C, Foxman B, et al. Mixed vaginitis-more than coinfection and with therapeutic implications. Curr Infect Dis Rep 2013;15(2):104.
14. Huh W, Ault KA, Chelmow D, et al. Use of primary high-risk human papillomavirus testing for cervical cancer screening: interim clinical guidance. J Low Genit Tract Dis 2015;19(2):91–6.
15. Palefsky JM. Human papillomavirus infections: epidemiology and disease associations. Available at: https://www.uptodate.com/contents/human-papillomavirus-infections-epidemiology-and-disease-associations?search=human-papillomavirus-uinfections-epidemiology-and-disease-associations&source=search_result&selectedTitle=1~150&usage_type=default&display_rank=1. Accessed March 13, 2018..
16. Silverberg MJ, Thorsen P, Lindenberg H, et al. Condyloma in pregnancy is strongly predictive of juvenile-onset recurrent respiratory papillomatosis. Obstet Gynecol 2003;101(4):645–52.
17. Carusi D. Treatment of vulvar and vaginal warts. 2017. Available at: https://www.uptodate.com/contents/treatment-of-vulvar-and-vaginal-warts?search=Treatment%20of%20vulvar%20and%20vaginal%20warts.&source=search_result&selectedTitle=1~150&usage_type=default&display_rank=1. Accessed March 13, 2018.
18. Albrecht, MA. Epidemiology, clinical manifestations, and diagnosis of genital herpes simplex virus infection. 2017. Available at: https://www.uptodate.com/contents/epidemiology-clinical-manifestations-and-diagnosis-of-genital-herpes-simplex-virus-infection?source=search_result&search=herpes%20simplex%20virus&selectedTitle=4~150. Accessed March 13, 2018.
19. Bernstein DI, Bellamy AR, Hook EW 3rd, et al. Epidemiology, clinical presentation, and antibody response to primary infection with herpes simplex virus type 1 and type 2 in young women. Clin Infect Dis 2013;56(3):344.
20. Sheffield JS, Hollie LM, Hill JB, et al. Acyclovir prophylaxis to prevent herpes simplex recurrence at delivery. Am J Obstet Gynecol 2003;102:1396–403.
21. Tully JG, Taylor-Robinson D, Cole RM, et al. A newly discovered mycoplasma in the human urogenital tract. Lancet 1981;1:1288.

22. Edouard S, Tissot-Dupont H, Dubourg G, et al. *Mycoplasma genitalium*, an agent of reemerging sexually transmitted infections. APMIS 2017. https://doi.org/10.11111/apm.12731.

23. Mobley V, Sena A. *Mycoplasma genitalium* infection in men and women. 2017. Available at: https://www.uptodate.com/contents/mycoplasma-genitalium-infection-in-men-and-women?search=Mycoplasma%20genitalium%20infection%20in%20men%20and%20women&source=search_result&selectedTitle=1~150&usage_type=default&display_rank=1. Accessed March 13, 2018.

24. Munson E, Wenten D, Jhansale S, et al. Expansion of comprehensive screening of male sexually transmitted infection clinic attendees with *Mycoplasma genitalium* and *Trichomonasa vaginalis* molecular assessment: a retrospective analysis. J Clin Microbiol 2017;55:321.

25. Cazanave C, Manhart LE, Bébéar C. *Mycoplasma genitalium*, an emerging sexually transmitted pathogen. Med Mal Infect 2012;42:381.

26. Donders GGG, Ruban K, Bellen G, et al. Mycoplasma/ureaplasma infection in pregnancy: to screen or not to screen. J Perinat Med 2017;45(5):505–15.

The Psychosocial and Clinical Well-Being of Women Living with Human Immunodeficiency Virus/AIDS

Safiya George Dalmida, PhD[a],*, Kyle R. Kraemer, MA[b],
Stephen Ungvary, MA[b], Elizabeth Di Valerio, BS[c],
Harold G. Koenig, MD[d,e], Marcia McDonnell Holstad, PhD[f]

KEYWORDS

- HIV/AIDS • Religion • Spirituality • Depression • Social support • Mental health

KEY POINTS

- Depression in women living with human immunodeficiency virus/AIDS is associated with poor adherence to treatment, and it negatively impacts quality of life.
- Spirituality/religiosity is important for many women living with human immunodeficiency virus/AIDS and is positively associated with coping, health practices, and health outcomes.
- In the present study, women living with human immunodeficiency virus/AIDS who reported depression had poorer health outcomes, greater perceived stress, and more negative religious coping behaviors.
- Religious attendance and religious coping significantly predicted depressive symptoms in women living with human immunodeficiency virus/AIDS .
- The role of religiosity in improving health outcomes in women living with human immunodeficiency virus/AIDS is highlighted.

INTRODUCTION

Owing to the success of highly active antiretroviral therapy (ART), human immunodeficiency virus (HIV) infection is now widely considered a chronic illness. Of the 1.2

[a] University of Alabama, Capstone College of Nursing, 650 University Boulevard, Tuscaloosa, AL 35487, USA; [b] Department of Psychology, University of Alabama, Box 870348, Tuscaloosa, AL 35487-0348, USA; [c] Department of Biological Sciences, University of Alabama, Box 870344, Tuscaloosa, AL 35487, USA; [d] Department of Psychiatry, Duke University Medical Center, 10 Duke Medicine Circle, Durham, NC 27710, USA; [e] Department of Medicine, King Abdulaziz University, Jeddah 22252, Saudi Arabia; [f] Emory University, Nell Hodgson Woodruff School of Nursing, 1520 Clifton Road, Atlanta, GA 30322, USA
* Corresponding author.
E-mail address: sfgeorge@ua.edu

Nurs Clin N Am 53 (2018) 203–225
https://doi.org/10.1016/j.cnur.2018.01.008
0029-6465/18/© 2018 Elsevier Inc. All rights reserved.

million people living with HIV/AIDS (PLWH) in the United States at the end of 2015, approximately one-quarter of these were women.[1] Despite the decrease in HIV diagnoses among women in recent years, more than 7000 received an HIV diagnosis in 2015.[2] Black/African American women are disproportionately affected by HIV, compared with women of other races/ethnicities, and account for more than 60% of women living with HIV/AIDS (WLWHA; compared with 17% each for white/Caucasian and Hispanic/Latina women).[2] WLWHA experience several challenges that may negatively impact psychosocial and clinical well-being.[3–12]

REVIEW OF THE LITERATURE
Depression and Human Immunodeficiency Virus

Depression is a major public health problem among people is duplicate of PLWH—particularly women and African Americans.[9,13–25] Depression rates are as high as 67% among WLWHA[19,24] and up to 64% among African American women with HIV.[26–28] Studies identified high rates of depression in HIV-positive African American women (43%) and in predominantly African American samples of PLWH (57%).[9–11,29,30] Yet, there are no known interventions that target major depression specifically in African American women with HIV.[26,27,31,32] African Americans have more difficulty accessing standard mental health care and may benefit less from it.[33–39] African American and Latina women living with HIV are less likely to receive adequate treatment for depression compared with Caucasian non-Hispanic women.[39–41] African Americans face the most severe burden of HIV and African American women represent 62% of HIV infections in women.[42] Depression in PLWH adversely affects adherence to ART,[17,43–47] immune function,[22] disease progression, comorbidity, mortality,[17,22,48–52] and quality of life.[10,20,21,40] Depression's negative effect on adherence is important because suboptimal adherence (<90%–95%) contributes to antiretroviral resistance and worse medical outcomes.[53–58]

Spirituality/Religion

Spirituality/religion is an important part of daily life for many African Americans (79%), Americans in the Southeast (69%-75%),[30,59,60] and PLWH (85%),[61] including African American WLWHA.[23] Among 2266 PLWH, 72% relied on their religious/spiritual resources when facing problems/difficulties, 86% identified as "religious" and 95% as "spiritual"; furthermore, African Americans reported significantly more religiosity than Caucasians.[61] Religiosity/spirituality may play a critical protective role in the mental well-being of Southern WLWHA[8–10,21,23] and may have an effect on mental health comparable with that of formal psychotherapy.[23] Our previous research[29] with WLWHA revealed that spirituality/religion is important in supporting their coping, health practices and health outcomes, fostering better mental health, treatment adherence, and CD4 T-cell count (an important marker of immune function). Findings of previous studies highlighted the role of spirituality and religious coping in improving depressive symptoms, ART adherence, CD4 cell count, and health-related quality of life (HRQOL) among HIV-positive women[9,10,29] and PLWH.[11,62] In research among WLWHA, including HIV-positive African American women, greater spirituality was significantly associated with fewer depressive symptoms,[9,11,21,23] better ART adherence, and improved immune function.[9,20,63] Despite this finding, few or no religious interventions exist to improve depression, adherence, and immune function in WLWHA.[17]

Human Immunodeficiency Virus Care and Clinical Outcomes

Up to 63% of patients with chronic medical conditions do not adhere to treatment,[64,65] resulting in an estimated cost of $300 billion per year.[66] Maintaining stable, functional wellness while living with HIV infection requires life-long and exceedingly high levels of adherence. Among PLWH, differential adherence is associated with a more rapid progression to AIDS and death,[55] but remains understudied,[54] although improvements of even 5% to 10% in adherence may lead to better biological outcomes.[53,57,67] ART is also important in HIV prevention. Lower or undetectable viral load (VL) resulting from optimal ART adherence is linked with a lower risk of HIV transmission.[68,69] Yet, only 30% of PLWH (28% of African Americans, 31% of Hispanics) in the United States attain adequate viral suppression and only 40% of PLWH are engaged in care.[70,71] The overall effectiveness of HIV treatment is severely undermined by attrition of patients across the HIV care continuum.[72]

To address the National HIV/AIDS Strategy and Healthy People 2020 HIV objectives, greater proportions of PLWH need to achieve each step across the HIV care continuum.[70] As such, PLWH should be (1) diagnosed, (2) linked to care, (3) engaged or retained in care (engaged is $\geq$1 documented CD4 count or VL) in a 12 month-period; retained is $\geq$2 documented CD4 count or VL in 12 a month-period, (4) prescribed ART, and (5) virally suppressed (VL of <200 copies/mL).

Linkage to and retention in HIV care is often worse among younger persons, females, and racial/ethnic minorities.[39,70,73–76] Poor engagement in HIV care and ART adherence are related to antiretroviral resistance, suboptimal CD4 count and VL,[76–78] and death,[78–80] and contribute to racial disparities in outcomes.[53–58,81] Current interventions have not been broadly effective in improving adherence or viral suppression or reaching HIV-positive African American women.[82,83] Supporting patient adherence to HIV care is key for optimizing health outcomes and functional wellness. Factors that negatively affect adherence to HIV treatment and care among PLWH include depression,[17,39–41,43–47] HIV stigma,[80,84] lack of social support,[40,41] and low motivation.[12,85,86] Therefore, tailored programs to enhance motivation and adherence offer great potential to mitigate barriers to maintaining stable health[87] and functional wellness.

This work describes the psychosocial well-being of WLWHA in the Southeastern United States and examines psychosocial factors that impact mental health, specifically level of depression, stress level, quality of life, and emotional well-being. The article also documents differences in clinical outcomes between WLWHA with symptoms of depression and WLWHA without depression.

METHODS
Participants and Procedures

A descriptive, cross-sectional study was conducted with a sample of WLWHA. Participants were recruited from an outpatient infectious disease clinic at a large university-affiliated health center and 2 AIDS service organizations in the Southeastern United States. Approval was obtained from the university's institutional review board and subjects were recruited using fliers that described the study purpose, procedures, eligibility criteria, and contained the contact information for study staff. Eligibility criteria required participants to be HIV positive, 18 years of age or older, able to speak and understand English, and mentally competent as determined by a score of 27 or greater on the Mini Mental Status Exam. The sample included 129 WLWHA. Each participant received $15 for participation.

Measures

Demographic
Information was collected using a 20-item form that solicited information about socio-economic status, age, race/ethnicity, gender, year of HIV diagnosis, approximate annual and monthly income, highest level of education completed, and employment/occupational status.

Religiousness
A modified version of the Brief Multidimensional Measure of Religiousness/Spirituality[88] assessed religious involvement and behavior and self-rated spirituality and religiousness. The Brief Multidimensional Measure of Religiousness/Spirituality items survey a variety of dimensions of religiosity, including daily spiritual experiences, meaning, values/beliefs, forgiveness, private religious practices, religious and spiritual coping, religious support, religious/spiritual history, commitment, organizational religiousness, religious preference, and overall self-ranking as a religious or spiritual person. Thirty-three of the original 38 items were used.

Religious coping
The short version of the Religious Coping Scale (RCOPE)[89] was used to assess religious coping. The Brief RCOPE is a 14 item scale that measures 2 dimensions: positive religious coping and negative religious coping, with 7 items each.[89] Participants rate their coping strategies using a 4-point rating scale from 1 (not at all) to 4 (a great deal). Positive religious coping items include strategies such as seeking spiritual support and benevolent reappraisals. The negative RCOPE contained items related to spiritual struggle such as, "I questioned God's love for me" and "I wondered whether God had abandoned me." Responses are summed to create subscale scores, with higher scores representing more frequent use of negative or positive religious coping. The Cronbach's alpha in this study for the negative RCOPE was 0.83 and for the positive RCOPE it was 0.90.

Perceived stress
The Perceived Stress Scale, which consists of 10 items, assessed the degree to which respondents found their lives unpredictable, uncontrollable, and overloaded. The Cronbach's alpha in this study was 0.85.

Depressive symptoms
The Center for Epidemiologic Studies Depression scale (CES-D) assessed symptoms of depression over the previous 7 days.[90] The scale consists of 20 items, scored on a 4-point scale from 0 (rarely) to 3 (most or all of the time). Scores of 16 or greater indicate a significant level of depression.[91] The scale reliability has been established and used successfully in PLWH.[92,93] The Cronbach alpha in this study was 0.90.

Social support
The Social Support Questionnaire–6[94] assessed satisfaction with social support via a 6-item abbreviated version of the 27-item Social Support Questionnaire. The items assessed the number of people who the individual feels he or she can turn to and the degree of satisfaction with the support available on a 6-point Likert scale (from very dissatisfied to very satisfied). The Social Support Questionnaire-6 has high internal reliability, with alphas from 0.90 to 0.93. The Cronbach alpha in the current study was 0.92.

Human immunodeficiency virus medication adherence

The Antiretroviral General Adherence Survey[95,96] measured adherence to HIV medications. The Antiretroviral General Adherence Survey is composed of 5 items that focus on the ease and ability of taking HIV medications as prescribed. Original reported Cronbach's alphas for the Antiretroviral General Adherence Survey in studies with both men living with HIV/AIDS and WLWHA were 0.74 and 0.80, respectively.[95,96]

Human immunodeficiency virus viral load

Participants provided a self-report of their most recent HIV VL: (a) undetectable at less than 50 copies/mL of blood, (b) undetectable at less than 400 copies/mL blood, (c) 400 to 1000 copies/mL blood, (d) greater than 1000 copies/mL blood, or (e) do not know/do not remember. This variable was then collapsed into 2 categories (undetectable and detectable).

CD4 cell count

CD4 cell counts were reported as the absolute number of CD4 T lymphocytes. These counts were assessed by self-report of the most recent laboratory results. The most recent laboratory date and study interview were often on the same day, but in some cases was up to 30 days earlier. With the participant's written consent, actual laboratory reports for CD4 cell count and HIV VL were obtained and reviewed.

Quality of life

HRQOL was measured using the RAND 36-Item Health Survey 1.0,[97] which assesses 8 dimensions of HRQOL life (physical functioning, role limitations owing to physical health, role limitations owing to emotional or personal problems, vitality [energy/fatigue], general health, emotional well-being, social functioning, and bodily pain).[97] Subscale response sets vary between scales. For example, for the physical functioning scale, responses occur on a 3-point scale that include 1 (yes, limited a lot), 2 (yes, limited a little), or 3 (no, not limited at all). The emotional well-being scale responses are a 6-point scale ranging from 1 (all of the time) to 6 (none of the time). A high score denotes a more favorable state of health. Composite scores for mental and physical HRQOL were used. The physical health composite score was composed of physical function, role limitations owing to physical health, bodily pain, and general health subscale scores.[97,98] The mental health composite score was composed of vitality (energy/fatigue), social functioning, role limitations owing to emotional or personal problems, and emotional well-being subscale scores.[97,98] For this study, the Cronbach alpha was 0.88 for the physical composite and 0.84 for the mental composite.

Statistical Analyses

Data were analyzed using SPSS statistical software package, version 23 (SPSS, Inc., Chicago, IL). For analysis, several variables were dichotomized, including prayer (at least once per week vs less than once per week), religious attendance (at least once per week vs less than once per week), race (black vs nonblack), education (at least high school vs less than high school), income (≥$21,000 per year vs <$21,000 per year), marriage (currently married or in a committed relationship vs widowed/separated/divorced/never married), religion (Christian vs non-Christian), and sexual orientation (heterosexual vs nonheterosexual). First, we used descriptive statistics to ascertain sample demographics. To determine the characteristics of depressed individuals, a series of one-way analyses of variance compared women with HIV who reported depressive symptoms on the CES-D (scores of ≥16) with women with HIV who scored less than 16. Pearson correlations were then used to determine potential covariates of depression and stress.

Multiple linear regression models determined the best predictors of depression, stress, mental quality of life, and emotional well-being. For depression, an additional logistic regression model distinguished the qualities that separated women with HIV who reported significant depressive symptoms (CES-D score of >15) from women without depression (CES-D score of <16). For each model, age, income, and education were entered into the model first. Next, measures of religion were entered into the model, including prayer, religious attendance, positive religious coping, and negative religious coping. Finally, social support satisfaction was added to the model to test whether social support mediated the relationship between religion and the variable of interest. Change in R^2 was assessed at each step, and β-values and their corresponding P values were used to determine which variables best predicted depression, stress, mental quality of life, and emotional well-being.

RESULTS
Sample Characteristics

Sample characteristics are given in **Table 1**. The majority of participants were African American/Black (n = 118 [92%]), heterosexual (n = 91 [72%]), had at least a high school education (n = 73 [58%]), and made less than $11,000/y (n = 89 [79%]). Most participants self-identified as religious (n = 119 [94%]) or spiritual (n = 121 [96%]), self-identified as Christian (n = 108 [92%]), prayed at least once per week (n = 106 [84%]), and attended church at least once each month (n = 97 [77%]). There was a high number of WLWHA with significant depressive symptoms (n = 79 [63%]).

Comparisons Between Women Living with Human Immunodeficiency Virus/AIDS with Depressive Symptoms versus Those Without Depressive Symptoms

On average, women who reported depressive symptoms had significantly worse outcomes on several measures (**Table 2**). Compared with nondepressed women, depressed women had significantly lower mean scores for social support satisfaction (P = .01; 4.99 vs 5.54), physical function (P = .03; 49.51 vs 60.62), physical quality of life (P<.01; 44.50 vs 60.41), physical role limitations (P<.01; 32.28 vs 50.91), general health (P<.001; 48.57 vs 61.30), HIV adherence (P<.01; 23.11 vs 26.53), and CD4 count (P = .01; 353.64 vs 696.86). Women with significant depressive symptoms reported higher perceived stress (P<.001; 21.52 vs 12.24), more negative religious coping (P<.001; 6.52 vs 2.96), and had a higher HIV VL (P = .02; 2.19 vs 0.88) compared with women who scored below the threshold of 16 on the CES-D.

Correlates of Depressive Symptoms

Pearson correlations revealed that social support satisfaction, prayer, and religious attendance were negatively correlated with stress and depressive symptoms, whereas negative religious coping was positively related to stress and depressive symptoms. Depressive symptoms were marginally associated with having less than a high school education and with being unmarried/uncommitted. Perceived stress was marginally associated with having an income of less than $21,000 per year and with identifying as nonheterosexual (**Table 3**).

Predictors of Threshold Depression

The logistic model of significant depressive symptoms (1 = CES-D ≥16; 0 = CES-D <16) is presented in **Table 4**. Specifically, block 1, which only included baseline demographics (age, income, education) predicted depression relatively poorly, Wald

Table 1
Sample characteristics

Variable	Mean	SD
Age (y)	45.00	7.24
Monthly income	613.07	815.44
Perceived total stress	18.16	7.82
Social support satisfaction	5.17	1.22
Quality of life: mental	48.51	10.54
CES-D depression	20.71	12.01
Quality of life: emotional	60.54	23.37
Religious coping: positive	17.27	4.40
Religious coping: negative	5.17	5.02
Years HIV positive	10.02	6.33
CD4 count	467.21	447.13

Variable	n	%
Race		
Black/African American	118	92.91
White/Caucasian	4	3.15
Asian/Pacific Islander	1	0.79
Native American/American Indian	1	0.79
Hispanic/Latino or Latina	1	0.79
Other	2	1.57
Education		
Less than high school	19	15.80
High school or GED	73	57.94
College or technical school	29	23.02
Graduate or professional school	5	3.97
Marital status		
Married	19	14.96
Separated/divorced/widowed	53	41.73
Never been married	36	28.35
Committed relationship	19	14.96
Income (US$)		
0–10,999	89	78.76
11,000–20,999	15	13.27
≥21,000	9	7.96
Religious affiliation		
Christian	108	92.31
Muslim or Buddhist	2	1.70
Belief in God-unspecified or other	6	5.13
Atheist or no belief in God	1	0.85
Religious self-rating		
Very/moderately religious	88	69.80
Slightly religious	31	24.60
Not religious at all	7	5.60

(continued on next page)

Table 1 (continued)		
Variable	n	%
Spiritual self-rating		
Very/moderately spiritual	94	74.60
Slightly spiritual	27	21.40
Not spiritual at all	5	4.00
Prayer		
More than once a day	62	49.20
Once a day	22	17.50
One to a few times a week	22	17.50
A few times a month	10	7.90
Never/rarely	10	8.00
Religious service attendance		
Every week or more often	57	45.30
Every month or so	40	31.80
Once or twice a year	22	17.50
Never	7	5.60
Depression status		
Depressed	79	63.2
Not depressed	46	36.8
Sexual orientation		
Straight/heterosexual	91	71.7
Gay/lesbian/homosexual	34	26.8

Abbreviations: CES-D, Center for Epidemiologic Studies Depression Scale; HIV, human immunodeficiency virus.

$\chi^2(3) = 6.38$, $P = .10$, although education individually did marginally predict less depression, Wald $\chi^2(1) = 3.39$, $P = .07$. Block 2, which included religious predictors, explained a significant proportion of the variance in depression, Wald $\chi^2(4) = 24.22$, $P<.01$, owing primarily to the effects of negative religious coping, Wald $\chi^2(1) = 11.04$, $P<.01$, and religious attendance, Wald $\chi^2(1) = 3.34$, $P = .07$. Including social support satisfaction in block 3 did not result in substantial changes from block 2 with regard to the effects of negative religious coping, Wald $\chi^2(1) = 10.12$, $P = .001$, or religious attendance, Wald $\chi^2(1) = 3.76$, $P = .05$.

Linear Regression Results

For the results of regression models of depression, stress, mental health quality of life, and emotional well-being (assessed as continuous variables), see **Table 5**. No significant contribution to the models emerged from block 1, when the demographic factors of age, income, and education were entered into the models first: stress, $F(3, 105) = 1.21$ ($P = .31$); mental quality of life, $F(3, 104) = 0.56$ ($P = .64$); depression, $F(3, 104) = 0.90$ ($P = .45$); emotional well-being, $F(3, 104) = 1.51$ ($P = .22$). Furthermore, age, income, and education did not individually predict any of the variables of interest, with the potential exception of emotional well-being, which was marginally predicted by education ($\beta = 0.17$; $P = .09$).

When measures of religion were entered into each model in block 2, these predictors together accounted for significant variance within stress, $F(4, 101) = 5.29$ ($P<.01$);

Table 2
Differences between depressed and nondepressed WLWHA

Variable	F	df	P	Not Depressed n	Mean	SD	Depressed n	Mean	SD
Age	0.20	1	123	.65	46	45.46	8.03	79	—	6.84
Monthly income	0.01	1	114	.91	40	622.73	543.60	76	605.53	934.99
Number of children	0.48	1	101	.49	37	2.89	1.91	66	3.67	6.65
Years living with HIV diagnosis	0.02	1	119	.90	45	10.07	6.62	76	9.91	6.27
Hours worked per week	2.19	1	114	.14	42	6.79	15.08	74	3.34	9.96
Social support satisfaction	6.26	1	122	.01	45	5.54	0.94	79	4.99	1.30
Physical function	4.92	1	123	.03	46	60.62	25.06	79	49.51	28.04
Physical composite QOL	17.19	1	123	.00	46	60.41	20.18	79	44.50	20.96
Physical role limitations subscale QOL	6.90	1	123	.01	46	50.91	40.72	79	32.28	36.72
Emotional role limitations subscale QOL	8.09	1	123	.01	46	60.87	43.49	79	38.82	40.80
Energy/fatigue/vitality QOL subscale	28.06	1	123	.00	46	62.17	19.51	79	44.24	17.49
Emotional well-being QOL subscale	66.44	1	123	.00	46	78.61	17.18	79	50.03	19.83
Social functioning QOL subscale	29.21	1	123	.00	46	80.71	23.38	79	53.16	29.59
Pain QOL Subscale	16.27	1	123	.00	46	68.8	25.67	79	47.66	29.66
AGAS (HIV adherence) total	8.20	1	100	.01	36	26.53	5.03	66	23.11	6.13
CD4 count	6.56	1	45	.01	14	696.86	633.79	33	353.64	291.91
Perceived stress total	60.55	1	123	.00	46	12.24	7.13	79	21.52	5.99
Mental composite QOL	39.95	1	123	.00	46	70.59	21.53	79	46.56	19.87
General health	12.35	1	123	.00	46	61.30	19.07	79	48.57	19.82
Positive religious coping	3.80	1	123	.05	46	18.26	4.41	79	16.68	4.33
Negative religious coping	16.23	1	123	.00	46	2.96	4.49	79	6.52	4.92
HIV viral load (log)	5.48	1	51	.02	16	0.88	1.78	37	2.19	1.91

Abbreviations: AGAS, Antiretroviral General Adherence Survey; HIV, human immunodeficiency virus; QOL, quality of life; SD, standard deviation; WLWHA, women living with HIV/AIDS.

depression, $F(4, 100) = 9.59$ ($P<.01$); mental health quality of life, $F(4, 100) = 2.94$ ($P = .02$); and emotional well-being, $F(4, 101) = 5.72$ ($P<.01$). Individual religious predictors demonstrated that religious attendance and negative religious coping contributed significantly to each model, with the exception of the model for mental quality of life, for which the effect of negative religious coping was only marginal ($\beta = -0.17$; $P = .09$). No other individual religious predictors made significant contributions beyond religious attendance and negative coping. Last, social support satisfaction was added to each model to test whether social support mediated the relationship between religion and the variables of interest. Although social support satisfaction contributed significantly to the prediction of depression, $F(1, 99) = 6.22$ ($P = .01$); stress, $F(1, 100) = 11.10$ ($P<.01$); mental quality of life, $F(1, 99) = 10.80$ ($P<.01$); and emotional well-being, $F(1, 99) = 8.93$ ($P<.01$), the degree to which religious attendance and negative religious coping predicted these factors remained relatively constant

Table 3

Correlations

Variable	Perceived Stress	QOL: Mental	QOL: Emotional	CES-D	Social Support Satisfaction	Religious Coping: Positive	Religious Coping: Negative	Prayer	Religious Attendance	Years HIV Positive	Age	Race (Black)	Income (High School)	Income <21K	Married or Committed Christian
Perceived Stress	1	—	—	—	—	—	—	—	—	—	—	—	—	—	—
QOL: mental	−.730[b]	1	—	—	—	—	—	—	—	—	—	—	—	—	—
QOL: Emotional	−.758[b]	.781[b]	1	—	—	—	—	—	—	—	—	—	—	—	—
depression (CES-D)	.722[b]	−.645[b]	−.732[b]	1	—	—	—	—	—	—	—	—	—	—	—
Social support satisfaction	−.289[b]	.339[b]	.324[b]	−.328[b]	1	—	—	—	—	—	—	—	—	—	—
Religious coping: positive	−0.067	0.107	.195[a]	−.160[c]	.184[a]	1	—	—	—	—	—	—	—	—	—
Religious coping: negative	.302[b]	−.187[a]	−.307[b]	.377[b]	−0.097	−0.064	1	—	—	—	—	—	—	—	—
Prayer	−.186[a]	.214[a]	.290[b]	−.265[b]	.163[c]	0.142	−.200[a]	1	—	—	—	—	—	—	—

Religious attendance	-.273[b]	.277[b]	.268[b]	-.280[b]	0.026	.263[b]	-0.039	.268[b]	1	—	—	—	—	—	—	—	—
Years HIV positive	-0.071	-0.029	0.038	-0.052	-0.056	0.066	0.057	-0.021	0.004	1	—	—	—	—	—	—	—
Age	0.008	-0.018	-0.004	0.066	-0.073	-0.038	-0.035	-0.079	0.1	0.05	1	—	—	—	—	—	—
Race (black)	0.014	0.018	0.044	0.004	.158[c]	-0.004	0.046	0.048	0.128	-0.113	-0.115	1	—	—	—	—	—
Education (high school)	-0.119	.164[c]	.223[a]	-.166[c]	.182[a]	.216[a]	-0.037	.241[b]	0.113	-0.046	-0.112	-0.031	1	—	—	—	—
Income (<$21K)	-0.159[c]	0.116	0.132	-0.118	-0.082	0.01	0.063	0.151	0.068	.212[a]	-0.02	-0.11	0.115	1	—	—	—
Married or committed	-0.056	0.094	0.143	-.157[c]	.196[a]	.247[b]	-0.032	-0.006	0.063	0.001	-.184[a]	0.113	0.132	-0.123	1	—	—
Christian	-0.031	-0.018	-0.013	-0.032	-0.019	0.11	-.157[c]	0.017	0.001	-0.054	-0.104	0.02	0.086	0.006	-0.073	1	—
Sexual orientation (heterosexual)	0.148[c]	-0.027	-0.144	0.150[c]	-0.139	-0.077	0.014	-0.133	-0.148[c]	0.027	0.144	-0.108	-0.192	-0.186[c]	0.026	-0.127	1

Abbreviations: CES-D, Center for Epidemiologic Studies Depression Scale; HIV, human immunodeficiency virus; QOL, quality of life.

[a] Less than .05.
[b] Less than .001.
[c] Less than .10.

Table 4
Predictors of depressive symptom status among WLWHA

DV	Model	Independent Variable	B	SE	Wald	df	P	Exp(B)
Depression	4	F(8,99) = 6.29, P<.001						
symptom		Step 1						0.03
category		Intercept	3.12	1.77	3.10	1	.08	22.67
		Age	−0.01	0.03	0.23	1	.63	0.99
		Income	−0.42	0.49	0.71	1	.40	0.66
		Education	−1.98	1.08	3.39	1	.07	0.14
		Step 2						
		Intercept	4.11	2.45	2.82	1	.09	61.09
		Age	−0.02	0.03	0.30	1	.59	0.98
		Income	−0.74	0.59	1.59	1	.21	0.47
		Education	−1.50	1.18	1.63	1	.20	0.22
		Prayer	−0.46	0.87	0.27	1	.60	0.63
		Religious attendance	−0.88	0.48	3.34	1	.07	0.41
		Religious coping: positive	−0.07	0.06	1.30	1	.25	0.93
		Religious coping: negative	0.19	0.06	11.04	1	.0008	1.22
		Step 3						
		Intercept	5.53	2.67	4.28	1	.038	251.73
		Age	−0.02	0.03	0.23	1	.635	0.98
		Income	−0.77	0.61	1.61	1	.204	0.46
		Education	−1.53	1.19	1.63	1	.202	0.22
		Prayer	−0.40	0.88	0.21	1	.651	0.67
		Religious attendance	−0.96	0.49	3.76	1	.052	0.38
		Religious coping: positive	−0.04	0.07	0.35	1	.554	0.96
		Religious coping: negative	0.19	0.06	10.16	1	.001	1.22
		Social support satisfaction	−0.38	0.27	2.05	1	.153	0.68

Abbreviations: DV, dependent variable; HIV, human immunodeficiency virus; SE, standard error; WLWHA, women living with human immunodeficiency virus/AIDS.

compared with the previous block. Thus, social support satisfaction did not mediate the relationship between religious behaviors and mental health.

DISCUSSION

This study examined differences in psychosocial health outcomes between depressed and nondepressed WLWHA and examined the factors that explained depressive symptoms, perceived stress, mental quality of life, and emotional well-being in a sample of 129, predominantly African American WLWHA. Sixty-three percent reported depressive symptoms, which is consistent with findings from other studies with depression rates as high as 67% among women living with HIV[19,24] and up to 64% among African American women with HIV.[26–28] Additionally, WLWHA with depressive symptoms in our sample reported significantly poorer health outcomes, including poorer HIV medication adherence, lower CD4 cell count, and poorer HRQOL. These findings are similar to other studies among PLWH and WLWHA,[29] which show that depression adversely affects HIV medication adherence,[17,19,43–47] immune function,[22] and quality of life.[10,20,21,40]

Table 5
Regression results: predictors of mental well-being factors

DV	Model	Independent Variable	B	SE	Beta	P	R^2	Delta R^2	Adjusted R^2
Perceived total stress	Model 1	$F_{(8,100)} = 4.89$, $P<.001$							
		Step 1					0.03	0.03	0.01
		Intercept	20.24	5.64	—	.00	—	—	—
		Age	0.02	0.11	0.02	.87	—	—	—
		Income	-2.88	1.96	-0.14	.14	—	—	—
		Education	-2.42	2.44	-0.10	.33	—	—	0.15
		Step 2					0.20	0.17	
		Intercept	18.42	6.33	—	.00	—	—	—
		Age	0.04	0.10	0.04	.66	—	—	—
		Income	-3.23	1.85	-0.16	.08	—	—	—
		Education	-0.50	2.36	-0.02	.83	—	—	—
		Prayer	-0.95	2.19	-0.04	.67	—	—	—
		Religious attendance	-4.18	1.55	-0.26	.01	—	—	—
		Religious coping: positive	-0.05	0.18	-0.02	.80	—	—	—
		Religious coping: negative	0.47	0.15	0.30	.00	—	—	0.22
		Step 3					0.28	0.08	
		Intercept	27.46	6.62	—	.00	—	—	—
		Age	0.05	0.10	0.04	.64	—	—	—
		Income	-3.56	1.77	-0.18	.05	—	—	—
		Education	-0.68	2.25	-0.03	.76	—	—	—
		Prayer	-0.75	2.09	-0.03	.72	—	—	—
		Religious attendance	-4.34	1.47	-0.27	.00	—	—	—
		Religious coping: positive	0.09	0.18	0.04	.63	—	—	—
		Religious coping: negative	0.44	0.14	0.27	.00	—	—	—
		Social support satisfaction	-2.11	0.63	-0.29	.00	—	—	—

(continued on next page)

Table 5
(continued)

DV	Model	Independent Variable	B	SE	Beta	P	R²	Delta R²	Adjusted R²
QOL: mental	Model 2	F(8,99) = 3.21, P = .003							
		Step 1					0.02	0.02	-0.01
		Intercept	62.18	16.79	—	.00	—	—	—
		Age	-0.22	0.32	-0.07	.48	—	—	—
		Income	4.70	5.71	0.08	.41	—	—	—
		Education	3.38	7.39	0.05	.65	—	—	—
		Step 2					0.12	0.10	0.06
		Intercept	62.30	19.46	—	.00	—	—	—
		Age	-0.30	0.31	-0.09	.34	—	—	—
		Income	4.97	5.61	0.09	.38	—	—	—
		Education	-1.79	7.40	-0.02	.81	—	—	—
		Prayer	2.80	6.66	0.04	.68	—	—	—
		Religious attendance	11.52	4.69	0.24	.02	—	—	—
		Religious coping: positive	0.24	0.55	0.04	.66	—	—	—
		Religious coping: negative	-0.76	0.44	-0.17	.09	—	—	—
		Step 3					0.21	0.09	0.14
		Intercept	32.24	20.70	—	.12	—	—	—
		Age	-0.28	0.30	-0.09	.35	—	—	—
		Income	6.09	5.36	0.10	.26	—	—	—
		Education	0.16	7.08	0.00	.98	—	—	—
		Prayer	1.82	6.36	0.03	.78	—	—	—
		Religious attendance	12.17	4.48	0.26	.01	—	—	—
		Religious coping: positive	-0.16	0.53	-0.03	.77	—	—	—
		Religious coping: negative	-0.64	0.42	-0.14	.13	—	—	—
		Social support satisfaction	6.47	1.97	0.31	.00	—	—	—

Depressive symptoms

Model 3

F(8,99) = 6.29, $P<.001$

	B	SE	β	p	R²	ΔR²	Adj. R²
Step 1							
Intercept	20.26	8.57	—	.02	0.03	0.03	0.00
Age	0.09	0.16	0.06	.57			
Income	−2.85	2.91	−0.10	.33			
Education	−3.57	3.77	−0.09	.35			
Step 2							
Intercept	19.59	8.92	—	.03	0.30	0.27	0.25
Age	0.13	0.14	0.08	.36			
Income	−3.71	2.57	−0.12	.15			
Education	0.52	3.39	0.01	.88			
Prayer	−2.22	3.05	−0.07	.47			
Religious attendance	−5.86	2.15	−0.24	.01			
Religious coping: positive	−0.29	0.25	−0.10	.25			
Religious coping: negative	0.950	0.202	0.406	.000			
Step 3							
Intercept	30.28	9.70	—	.00	0.34	0.04	0.28
Age	0.13	0.14	0.08	.37			
Income	−4.11	2.51	−0.14	.10			
Education	−0.17	3.32	0.00	.96			
Prayer	−1.87	2.98	−0.06	.53			
Religious attendance	−6.09	2.10	−0.25	.00			
Religious coping: positive	−0.15	0.25	−0.05	.55			
Religious coping: negative	0.905	0.198	0.387	.000			
Social support satisfaction	−2.30	0.92	−0.21	.01			

(continued on next page)

Table 5
(continued)

DV	Model	Independent Variable	B	SE	Beta	P	R²	Delta R²	Adjusted R²
QOL: emotional well-being	Model 4	F(8,99) = 4.93, P<.001							
		Step 1					0.042	0.042	0.014
		Intercept	48.69	16.76	—	.00	—	—	—
		Age	−0.01	0.32	0.00	.97	—	—	—
		Income	5.77	5.70	0.10	.31	—	—	—
		Education	12.77	7.38	0.17	.09	—	—	—
		Step 2					0.22	0.18	0.17
		Intercept	42.60	18.53	—	.02	—	—	—
		Age	−0.05	0.30	−0.02	.86	—	—	—
		Income	6.52	5.34	0.11	.23	—	—	—
		Education	5.39	7.04	0.07	.45	—	—	—
		Prayer	7.85	6.34	.12	.22	—	—	—
		Religious attendance	9.03	4.46	0.19	.05	—	—	—
		Religious coping: positive	0.61	0.52	0.11	.24	—	—	—
		Religious coping: negative	−1.32	0.42	−0.29	.00	—	—	—
		Step 3					0.29	0.06	0.23
		Intercept	16.35	19.88	—	.41	—	—	—
		Age	−0.04	0.28	−0.01	.90	—	—	—
		Income	7.49	5.15	0.13	.15	—	—	—
		Education	7.09	6.80	0.09	.30	—	—	—
		Prayer	6.99	6.11	0.10	.26	—	—	—
		Religious attendance	9.59	4.30	0.20	.03	—	—	—
		Religious coping: positive	0.27	0.51	0.05	.60	—	—	—
		Religious coping: negative	−1.22	0.41	−0.26	.00	—	—	—
		Social support satisfaction	5.65	1.89	0.26	.00	—	—	—

Abbreviations: DV, dependent variable; QOL, quality of life; SE, standard error.

In this study, WLWHA with depressive symptoms reported greater perceived stress and negative religious coping, and had lower social support satisfaction compared with WLWHA without depressive symptoms. Religious attendance and negative religious coping explained a significant amount of variance in depression, perceived stress, mental quality of health, and emotional well-being. The odds of being depressed were significantly higher among women who reported higher negative religious coping. The likelihood of experiencing depression was marginally lower in WLWHA who reported higher religious attendance. Being part of a religious community may confer considerable psychological benefit, particularly if that community is supportive rather than stigmatizing. These findings are consistent with those of other studies among WLWHA that have reported higher levels of spirituality associated with fewer depressive symptoms,[9,11,21,23] and better ART adherence and immune function.[9,20,63] In this study, social support did not mediate the relationship between religious coping or religious attendance and depressive symptoms. The literature contains mixed findings regarding whether or not social support mediates the link between spirituality and depression in PLWH/WLWHA.

The majority of participants (92%) in this study identified as Christian and a large proportion described themselves as moderately or very religious (70%) or moderately or very spiritual (75%). These religious demographics are similar to those of other studies in the Southeastern United States (which is often referred to as the "Bible Belt") among PLWH,[61] including African American WLWHA.[23] These rates are also similar for African Americans (79%) and Americans more generally in the Southeast (69%-75%).[30,59,60] Therefore, these results are best generalizable to WLWHA who identify as spiritual or religious.

SUMMARY

High rates of depressive symptoms were present and negatively associated with health outcomes. Religious involvement (particularly religious coping) was related to the severity of depressive symptoms, perceived stress, quality of life, and emotional well-being. Social support, although associated with these mental health outcomes, did not seem to moderate these relationships. These findings underscore the need for nurses and other health care providers to regularly screen WLWHA for and adequately treat depression. It is also important for nurses and physicians to collaborate with mental health providers, social workers, and pastoral care counselors in the care of WLWHA. This measure could help to address WLWHA's mental, social, and spiritual needs, and potentially optimize their HIV-related outcomes.

REFERENCES

1. Centers for Disease Control and Prevention (CDC). HIV surveillance report, 2015, vol. 27. Centers for Disease Control and Prevention; 2016.

2. Centers for Disease Control and Prevention (CDC). HIV among women. Available at: https://www.cdc.gov/hiv/group/gender/women/index.html#refb. Accessed December 1, 2017.

3. Beres LK, Narasimhan M, Robinson J, et al. Non-specialist psychosocial support interventions for women living with HIV: a systematic review. AIDS Care 2017; 29(9):1079–87.

4. Brown MJ, Serovich JM, Kimberly JA, et al. Psychological reactance and HIV-related stigma among women living with HIV. AIDS Care 2016;28(6): 745–9.

5. Rubtsova AA, Kempf M-C, Taylor TN, et al. Healthy aging in older women living with HIV infection: a systematic review of psychosocial factors. Curr HIV/AIDS Rep 2017;14(1):17–30.

6. Kelso-Chichetto NE, Okafor CN, Cook RL, et al. Association between depressive symptom patterns and clinical profiles among persons living with HIV. AIDS Behav 2017. [Epub ahead of print].

7. Illangasekare SL, Burke JG, Chander G, et al. Among women living with the substance abuse, violence, and HIV/AIDS syndemic: a qualitative exploration. Womens Health Issues 2014;24(5):551–7.

8. Dalmida SG. Spirituality, mental health, physical health, and health-related quality of life among women with HIV/AIDS: integrating spirituality into mental health care. Issues Ment Health Nurs 2006;27(2):185–98.

9. Dalmida SG, Holstad MM, Diiorio C, et al. Spiritual well-being, depressive symptoms, and immune status among women living with HIV/AIDS. Womens Health 2009;49(2–3):119–43.

10. Dalmida SG, Holstad MM, Diiorio C, et al. Spiritual well-being and health-related quality of life among African-American women with HIV/AIDS. Appl Res Qual Life 2011;6(2):139–57.

11. Dalmida SG, Koenig HG, Holstad MM, et al. The psychological well-being of people living with HIV/AIDS and the role of religious coping and social support. Int J Psychiatry Med 2013;46(1):57–83.

12. Holstad M, Spangler S, Higgins M, et al. Psychosocial characteristics associated with both antiretroviral therapy adherence and risk behaviors in women living with HIV. AIDS Behav 2016;20(5):1084–96.

13. Lopes M, Olfson M, Rabkin J, et al. Gender, HIV status, and psychiatric disorders: results from the National Epidemiologic Survey on Alcohol and Related Conditions. J Clin Psychiatry 2012;73(3):384–91.

14. Tedaldi EM, van den Berg-Wolf M, Richardson J, et al. Sadness in the SUN: using computerized screening to analyze correlates of depression and adherence in HIV-infected adults in the United States. AIDS Patient Care STDS 2012;26(12):718–29.

15. Hartzell JD, Janke IE, Weintrob AC. Impact of depression on HIV outcomes in the HAART era. J Antimicrob Chemother 2008;62(2):246–55.

16. Eller LS, Bunch EH, Wantland DJ, et al. Prevalence, correlates, and self-management of HIV-related depressive symptoms. AIDS Care 2010;22(9):1159–70.

17. Sherr L, Clucas C, Harding R, et al. HIV and depression–a systematic review of interventions. Psychol Health Med 2011;16(5):493–527.

18. Lopez AD, Murray CC. The global burden of disease, 1990-2020. Nat Med 1998;4(11):1241–3.

19. Cook JA, Grey D, Burke-Miller J, et al. Effects of treated and untreated depressive symptoms on highly active antiretroviral therapy use in a US multi-site cohort of HIV-positive women. AIDS Care 2006;18(2):93–100.

20. Dalmida SG. Relationships among spirituality, depression, immune status, and health-related quality of life in women with HIV. ProQuest; 2006.

21. George Dalmida S. Psychosocial and spiritual factors and depression among African-Americans living with HIV/AIDS. Paper presented at: Sigma Theta Tau International's 22nd International Nursing Research Congress. Cancun (Mexico), November 14, 2017.

22. Ickovics JR, Hamburger ME, Vlahov D, et al. Mortality, CD4 cell count decline, and depressive symptoms among HIV-seropositive women: longitudinal analysis from the HIV Epidemiology Research Study. JAMA 2001;285(11):1466–74.

23. Braxton ND, Lang DL, M Sales J, et al. The role of spirituality in sustaining the psychological well-being of HIV-positive black women. Womens Health 2007; 46(2–3):113–29.

24. Cook JA, Grey D, Burke J, et al. Depressive symptoms and AIDS-related mortality among a multisite cohort of HIV-positive women. Am J Public Health 2004;94(7): 1133–40.

25. Jones DJ, Beach SR, Forehand R, et al. Self-reported health in HIV-positive African American women: the role of family stress and depressive symptoms. J Behav Med 2003;26(6):577–99.

26. Logie C, James L, Tharao W, et al. Associations between HIV-related stigma, racial discrimination, gender discrimination, and depression among HIV-positive African, Caribbean, and Black women in Ontario, Canada. AIDS Patient Care STDS 2013; 27(2):114–22.

27. Simbayi LC, Kalichman S, Strebel A, et al. Internalized stigma, discrimination, and depression among men and women living with HIV/AIDS in Cape Town, South Africa. Soc Sci Med 2007;64(9):1823–31.

28. Field W, Kruger C. The effect of an art psychotherapy intervention on levels of depression and health locus of control orientations experienced by black women living with HIV. S Afr J Psychol 2008;38:467–78.

29. Dalmida SG, Holstad MM, Dilorio C, et al. The meaning and use of spirituality among African American women living with HIV/AIDS. West J Nurs Res 2012; 34(6):736–65.

30. Lewinsohn P, Clarke G, Hoberman HM. The coping with depression course: review and future directions. Can J Behav Sci 1989;21:470–93.

31. Moneyham L, Sowell R, Seals B, et al. Depressive symptoms among African American women with HIV disease. Res Theory Nurs Pract 2000;14(1):9–39.

32. Johnson SD, Cunningham-Williams RM, Cottler LB. A tripartite of HIV-risk for African American women: the intersection of drug use, violence, and depression. Drug Alcohol Depend 2003;70(2):169–75.

33. Himelhoch S, Josephs JS, Chander G, et al. Use of outpatient mental health services and psychotropic medications among HIV-infected patients in a multisite, multistate study. Gen Hosp Psychiatry 2009;31(6):538–45.

34. Himelhoch S, Mohr D, Maxfield J, et al. Feasibility of telephone-based cognitive behavioral therapy targeting major depression among urban dwelling African-American people with co-occurring HIV. Psychol Health Med 2011; 16(2):156–65.

35. Horrell SCV. Effectiveness of cognitive-behavioral therapy with adult ethnic minority clients: a review. Prof Psychol Res Pr 2008;39(2):160–8.

36. La Roche MJ, Christopher MS. Changing paradigms from empirically supported treatment to evidence-based practice: a cultural perspective. Professional Psychology: Research and Practice 2009;40(4):396.

37. Hall GCN. Psychotherapy research with ethnic minorities: empirical, ethical, and conceptual issues. J Consult Clin Psychol 2001;69(3):502.

38. Miranda J, Azocar F, Organista KC, et al. Treatment of depression among impoverished primary care patients from ethnic minority groups. Psychiatr Serv 2003; 54(2):219–25.

39. Cook JA, Burke-Miller JK, Grey DD, et al. Do HIV-positive women receive depression treatment that meets best practice guidelines? AIDS Behav 2014;18(6): 1094–102.

40. Dyer TP, Stein JA, Rice E, et al. Predicting depression in mothers with and without HIV: the role of social support and family dynamics. AIDS Behav 2012;16(8): 2198–208.

41. Vyavaharkar M, Moneyham L, Corwin S, et al. HIV-disclosure, social support, and depression among HIV-infected African American women living in the rural Southeastern United States. AIDS Educ Prev 2011;23(1):78–90.

42. Centers for Disease Control and Prevention. Social determinants of health among adults with diagnosed HIV infection in 20 states, the District of Columbia, and Puerto Rico, 2010. HIV Surveillance Supplemental Report 2014, Vol. 19. Atlanta (GA): Centers for Disease Control and Prevention; 2014.

43. Gonzalez JS, Batchelder AW, Psaros C, et al. Depression and HIV/AIDS treatment nonadherence: a review and meta-analysis. J Acquir Immune Defic Syndr 2011; 58(2):181–7.

44. Gonzalez JS, Psaros C, Batchelder A, et al. Clinician-assessed depression and HAART adherence in HIV-infected individuals in methadone maintenance treatment. Ann Behav Med 2011;42(1):120–6.

45. Harding R, Lampe FC, Norwood S, et al. Symptoms are highly prevalent among HIV outpatients and associated with poor adherence and unprotected sexual intercourse. Sex Transm Infect 2010;86(7):520–4.

46. Safren SA, Otto MW, Worth JL. Life-steps: applying cognitive behavioral therapy to HIV medication adherence. Cogn Behav Pract 1999;6(4):332–41.

47. Safren SA, Otto MW, Worth JL, et al. Two strategies to increase adherence to HIV antiretroviral medication: life-steps and medication monitoring. Behav Res Ther 2001;39(10):1151–62.

48. Fairfield KM, Libman H, Davis RB, et al. Delays in protease inhibitor use in clinical practice. J Gen Intern Med 1999;14(7):395–401.

49. Leserman J. HIV disease progression: depression, stress, and possible mechanisms. Biol Psychiatry 2003;54(3):295–306.

50. Freeman SM. Cognitive behavioral therapy in advanced practice nursing: an overview. Topics in Advanced Practice Nursing e-Journal 2006;6(3).

51. Leserman J, Petitto J, Gu H, et al. Progression to AIDS, a clinical AIDS condition and mortality: psychosocial and physiological predictors. Psychol Med 2002; 32(06):1059–73.

52. Beck JS, Reilly C. Nurses integrate cognitive therapy treatment into primary care. Description of clinical application of a pilot programme. Topics in Advanced Practice Nursing e-Journal 2006;6(3).

53. Bangsberg DR, Perry S, Charlebois ED, et al. Non-adherence to highly active antiretroviral therapy predicts progression to AIDS. AIDS 2001;15(9):1181–3.

54. Gardner EM, Sharma S, Peng G, et al. Differential adherence to combination antiretroviral therapy is associated with virological failure with resistance. AIDS 2008;22(1):75–82.

55. Mannheimer S, Thackeray L, Huppler Hullsiek K, et al. A randomized comparison of two instruments for measuring self-reported antiretroviral adherence. AIDS Care 2008;20(2):161–9.

56. Montaner JS, Reiss P, Cooper D, et al. A randomized, double-blind trial comparing combinations of nevirapine, didanosine, and zidovudine for HIV-infected patients: the INCAS Trial. Italy, The Netherlands, Canada and Australia Study. JAMA 1998;279(12):930–7.

57. Paterson DL, Swindells S, Mohr J, et al. Adherence to protease inhibitor therapy and outcomes in patients with HIV infection. Ann Intern Med 2000;133(1):21–30.

58. Stansell J, Holtzer C, Mayer S, et al. Factors affecting treatment outcomes in a medication event monitoring system. Retroviruses and opportunistic infections. Chicago (IL); 2001.

59. National Collaborating Centre for Mental Health. The treatment and management of depression in adults. National Institute for Health and Clinical Excellence (NICE). Clinical guideline no. 90. Leicester (UK): British Psychological Society; 2010.

60. Bradley NG, Lux LJ, Gartlehner G. Primary care depression guidelines and treatment resistant depression: variations on an important but understudied theme. 2012.

61. Lorenz KA, Hays RD, Shapiro MF, et al. Religiousness and spirituality among HIV-infected Americans. J Palliat Med 2005;8(4):774–81.

62. Hollon SD, Shaw BF. Group cognitive therapy for depressed patients. In: Beck AT, Rush AJ, Shaw BF, et al, editors. Cognitive therapy of depression. New York: Guilford Press; 1979. p. 328–53.

63. George Dalmida S. Spiritual, Religious and Psychosocial Correlates of Adherence Among African-American HIV-Positive Outpatients. Paper presented at: Sigma Theta Tau International's 22nd International Nursing Research Congress. Cancun (Mexico), November 14, 2017.

64. Rivet Amico K. A situated-Information Motivation Behavioral Skills Model of Care Initiation and Maintenance (sIMB-CIM): an IMB model based approach to understanding and intervening in engagement in care for chronic medical conditions. J Health Psychol 2011;16(7):1071–81.

65. Dunbar-Jacob J, Mortimer-Stephens M. Treatment adherence in chronic disease. J Clin Epidemiol 2001;54(12):S57–60.

66. DiMatteo MR. Variations in patients' adherence to medical recommendations: a quantitative review of 50 years of research. Med Care 2004;42(3):200–9.

67. Liu H, Miller LG, Hays RD, et al. Repeated measures longitudinal analyses of HIV virologic response as a function of percent adherence, dose timing, genotypic sensitivity, and other factors. J Acquir Immune Defic Syndr 2006;41(3):315–22.

68. Eaton JW, Johnson LF, Salomon JA, et al. HIV treatment as prevention: systematic comparison of mathematical models of the potential impact of antiretroviral therapy on HIV incidence in South Africa. PLoS Med 2012;9(7):e1001245.

69. Nguyen VK, Bajos N, Dubois-Arber F, et al. Remedicalizing an epidemic: from HIV treatment as prevention to HIV treatment is prevention. AIDS 2011;25(3):291–3.

70. Centers for Disease Control and Prevention (CDC). CDC fact sheet: HIV in the United States: the stages of care. Atlanta (GA): Centers for Disease Control and Prevention; 2014.

71. Centers for Disease Control and Prevention (CDC). CDC fact sheet. HIV in the United States: the stages of care. vol. 21. Atlanta (GA): Centers for Disease Control and Prevention; 2012.

72. McNairy ML, El-Sadr WM. The HIV care continuum: no partial credit given. AIDS 2012;26(14):1735–8.

73. Hall HI, Gray KM, Tang T, et al. Retention in care of adults and adolescents living with HIV in 13 U.S. areas. J Acquir Immune Defic Syndr 2012;60(1):77–82.

74. Rebeiro P, Althoff KN, Buchacz K, et al, North American AIDS Cohort Collaboration on Research and Design. Retention among North American HIV-infected

persons in clinical care, 2000-2008. J Acquir Immune Defic Syndr 2013;62(3): 356–62.

75. Ulett KB, Willig JH, Lin H-Y, et al. The therapeutic implications of timely linkage and early retention in HIV care. AIDS Patient Care STDS 2009;23(1):41–9.

76. Horstmann E, Brown J, Islam F, et al. Retaining HIV-infected patients in care: where are we? Where do we go from here? Clin Infect Dis 2010;50(5):752–61.

77. Robbins GK, Daniels B, Zheng H, et al. Predictors of antiretroviral treatment failure in an urban HIV clinic. J Acquir Immune Defic Syndr 2007;44(1):30–7.

78. Giordano TP, Gifford AL, White AC Jr, et al. Retention in care: a challenge to survival with HIV infection. Clin Infect Dis 2007;44(11):1493–9.

79. Park WB, Choe PG, Kim SH, et al. One-year adherence to clinic visits after highly active antiretroviral therapy: a predictor of clinical progress in HIV patients. J Intern Med 2007;261(3):268–75.

80. Turan B, Smith W, Cohen MH, et al. Mechanisms for the negative effects of internalized HIV-related stigma on antiretroviral therapy adherence in women: the mediating roles of social isolation and depression. J Acquir Immune Defic Syndr 2016;72(2):198–205.

81. Mugavero MJ, Amico KR, Horn T, et al. The state of engagement in HIV care in the United States: from cascade to continuum to control. Clin Infect Dis 2013;57(8): 1164–71.

82. Simoni JM, Pearson CR, Pantalone DW, et al. Efficacy of interventions in improving highly active antiretroviral therapy adherence and HIV-1 RNA viral load: a meta-analytic review of randomized controlled trials. J Acquir Immune Defic Syndr 2006;43(Suppl 1):S23.

83. de Bruin M, Viechtbauer W, Schaalma HP, et al. Standard care impact on effects of highly active antiretroviral therapy adherence interventions: a meta-analysis of randomized controlled trials. Arch Intern Med 2010;170(3):240–50.

84. Katz IT, Ryu AE, Onuegbu AG, et al. Impact of HIV-related stigma on treatment adherence: systematic review and meta-synthesis. J Int AIDS Soc 2013; 16(3 Suppl 2):18640.

85. Holstad MM, DiIorio C, Kelley ME, et al. Group motivational interviewing to promote adherence to antiretroviral medications and risk reduction behaviors in HIV infected women. AIDS Behav 2011;15(5):885–96.

86. Holstad MM, DiIorio C, Magowe MK. Motivating HIV positive women to adhere to antiretroviral therapy and risk reduction behavior: the KHARMA Project. Online J Issues Nurs 2006;11(1):5.

87. Teyhen DS, Aldag M, Centola D, et al. Incentives to create and sustain healthy behaviors: technology solutions and research needs. Mil Med 2014;179(12): 1419–31.

88. Abeles R, Ellison C, George L, et al. Multidimensional measurement of religiousness/spirituality for use in health research: a report of the Fetzer Institute/National Institute on Aging Working Group. In: Fetzer Institute, National Institute on Aging, editors. Kalamazoo (MI): Fetzer Institute; 1999. Available at: http://fetzer.org/sites/default/files/images/resources/attachment/%5Bcurrent-date%3Atiny%5D/Multidimensional_Measurement_of_Religousness_Spirituality.pdf.

89. Pargament KI, Smith BW, Koenig HG, et al. Patterns of positive and negative religious coping with major life stressors. J Sci Study Relig 1998;37(4):10–24.

90. Radloff LS, Locke BZ. The community mental health assessment survey and CES-D scale. In: Weissman MM, Meyers JK, editors. Community surveys of

psychiatric disorders. New Brunswick (NJ): Rutgers University Press; 1986. p. 177–87.

91. Radloff LS. The CES-D scale: a self-report depression scale for research in the general population. Appl Psychol Meas 1977;1(3):385–401.

92. Miles MS, Burchinal P, Holditch-Davis D, et al. Personal, family, and health-related correlates of depressive symptoms in mothers with HIV. J Fam Psychol 1997; 11(1):23.

93. Vedhara K, Schifitto G, McDermott M. Disease progression in HIV-positive women with moderate to severe immunosuppression: the role of depression. Dana consortium on therapy for HIV dementia and related cognitive disorders. Behav Med 1999;25(1):43–7.

94. Sarason IG, Sarason BR, Shearin EN, et al. A brief measure of social support: practical and theoretical implications. J Soc Pers Relat 1987;4(4):497–510.

95. Holstad MK, Pace JC, De AK, et al. Factors associated with adherence to antiretroviral therapy. J Assoc Nurses AIDS Care 2006;17(2):4–15.

96. Holstad MM, Foster V, Diiorio C, et al. An examination of the psychometric properties of the Antiretroviral General Adherence Scale (AGAS) in two samples of HIV-infected individuals. J Assoc Nurses AIDS Care 2010;21(2):162–72.

97. Hays RD, Sherbourne CD, Mazel RM. The RAND 36-item health survey 1.0. Health Econ 1993;2(3):217–27.

98. McHorney CA, Ware JJ, Raczek AE. The MOS 36-item short-form health survey (SF-36): II. psychometric and clinical tests of validity in measuring physical and mental health constructs. Med Care 1993;31:247–63.

Health Care of Sexual Minority Women

Susan Jo Roberts, DNSc, ANP

KEYWORDS

- Sexual minority women • Lesbians • Health promotion

KEY POINTS

- Knowledge about the health care of sexual minority women has been slowly accumulating over the last 3 decades.
- Sexual minority women have been heard when they speak up about their identity and their need to be included in the health care system.
- Sexual minority women have been heard in their need to know how health for sexual minority women is different than that of other women.
- Activists have been successful in engaging with the government to encourage inclusion of questions about sexual identity/behaviors on state and federal health questionnaires.
- These data have provided valuable information and comparisons with other groups of women.

Knowledge about the health care of sexual minority women (SMW) has been slowly accumulating over the last 3 decades. Owing to societal changes, SMW have been heard when they speak up about their identity, their need to be included in the health care system, and their need to know how health for SMW is different than that of other women. Activists have been successful in engaging with the government to encourage inclusion of questions about sexual identity/behaviors on state and federal health questionnaires that have provided valuable information and comparisons with other groups of women (**Box 1** provides definitions of terms).

The Institute of Medicine report,[1] *The Health of Lesbian, Gay, Bisexual and Transgender People: Building a Foundation for Better Understanding*, was critical in raising awareness to the lack of data on health care and requesting the funding needed to support research. Several presentations and books are available for providers to read that may assist when caring for this population (**Boxes 2–4**). This article reviews existing information on the health care needs of SMW: (1) factors in seeking care in health care settings, (2) specific risk factors and health care problems of SMW, and (3) recommendations for caring for SMW.

The author has no commercial or financial conflicts of interest or any funding sources.
School of Nursing, Northeastern University, 360 Huntington Avenue, Boston, MA 02115, USA
E-mail address: s.roberts@neu.edu

Nurs Clin N Am 53 (2018) 227–239
https://doi.org/10.1016/j.cnur.2018.01.009
0029-6465/18/© 2018 Elsevier Inc. All rights reserved.

Box 1
Definitions

- Sexual minority women—Lesbian, bisexual, or queer women.
- Lesbian—Women who identify as having primary sexual and loving relationships with women.
- Bisexual women—Women who identify as having sexual and loving relationships with both men and women.
- Women who have sex with women—Women who have sex with women and may identify themselves as lesbian, bisexual, or heterosexual.

FACTORS IN SEEKING CARE IN HEALTH CARE SETTINGS
The Patient–Provider Relationship

Early studies focused on the relationship between SMW and health care providers, and found that lesbians had negative experiences in health care encounters, and that nurses and physicians held negative attitudes toward them. Lesbians also reported fear that the quality of care would be negatively affected if they disclosed their sexuality and were therefore hesitant to disclose.[2,3] More recent studies have found higher rates of disclosure to providers, a change that most likely reflects increased comfort of SMW and providers owing to societal changes that have increased the visibility and acceptability of SMW in society.[4,5] A recent study found that 90% of individuals would not refuse to respond to inquiries about sexual orientation in the emergency room, but 80% of clinicians would not ask because they thought that patients would be offended.[6] These data clarify that patients are comfortable sharing information about their sexual behaviors/identity, but providers need to know and be comfortable in asking about those items.

The rights of same sex partners/spouses in hospitals, emergency rooms, delivery rooms, nursing homes, and palliative care units have improved over the past 2 decades, but providers may need to question their institutional policies regarding these rights. SMW need to be encouraged to enact legal paperwork so that their partners will have the right to be their medical power of attorney and/or health care proxy if needed. It is particularly important for the sexual minority community to have up-to-date

---

Box 2
Resources for clinicians

- Clunis DM, Green GE. The Lesbian Parenting Book: a guide to creating families and raising children. 2nd edition. New York: Seal Press; 2003.
- Eckstrand KL, Ehrenfield JM. Lesbian, gay, bisexual and transgender healthcare: a clinical guide to prevention. Switzerland: Springer International Publishing; 2016.
- Gay & Lesbian Medical Association (GLMA). Guidelines for care of lesbian, gay, bisexual and transgender patients. Available at: www.glma.org.
- Human Rights Campaign. Available at: http://www.hrc.org.
- Institute of Medicine. The health of lesbian, gay, bisexual and transgender people: building a foundation for better understanding. Washington, DC: National Academies Press; 2011.
- Makadon HJ, Mayer KH, Potter J, et al. The Fenway Guide to lesbian, gay, bisexual and transgender health. 2nd edition. Philadelphia: American College of Physicians; 2015.

Box 3
Specific clinical strategies necessary for optimal care of SMW

- Clinical forms and educational materials should be gender neutral (partner/spouse not husband).

- Ask all patients, "Are you having sex attraction or relationships with men, women, or both?"

- If currently having sex with only women, what was the past sexual history with men?

- If having sex with women, how comfortable is the patient in discussing this partner with family and coworkers, or in social settings?

- Screen for cancer, human immunodeficiency virus, and other sexually transmitted infections, following published guidelines.

- Focus interventions for obesity/overweight on becoming healthier rather than having a normal body mass index.

- Recommendation for childbirth and other educational forums that include other SMW and are sensitive to SMW.

- Determine if medical power of attorney and health care proxy documents are up to date.

- Availability and contact information for SMW sensitive providers or groups to assist SMW who are anxious or depressed regarding their sexual orientation.

- Screen for adverse childhood experiences and, if positive, ask how it has affected their life.

- Referrals for subspecialties that are SMW friendly and supportive.

Abbreviation: SMW, sexual minority women.

---

paperwork, and providers should clarify with the patient on every visit whether any of expectations or paperwork have changed.

Physical Examination, Cancer, and Sexually Transmitted Infection Screening

Early surveys also found that fewer than 50% of lesbians had an annual physical examination, and most sought care only when a problem arose. This lack of accessing services was due to their fear that telling providers about their sexuality would negatively affect their care. Results of a more recent survey demonstrated increased use of routine physicals.[5] Lesbians prefer a female and lesbian provider, and frequently use "alternative" providers, such as acupuncturists, massage therapists, and nonphysician health care providers.[3,7]

A metaanalysis that adjusted data from early lesbian surveys for comparison with the National Health Interview Survey found that lesbians had lower rates of pap smears than women in general.[8] More recent studies have found increased rates of

---

Box 4
Specific health concerns more frequently found in sexual minority women

- Obesity/overweight

- Tobacco use

- Alcohol abuse

- Mental health problems; especially anxiety and depression

- Childhood sexual abuse

pap smear screening, but the rate is still lower than national guidelines and heterosexual comparison groups.[5,9] This lower rate of screening was thought to be of less concern because of a belief that the incidence of cervical dysplasia was very low among women who did not have sex with men, and therefore they thought they did not need routine screening. However, research findings demonstrate that human papillomavirus infection is found in 13% to 30% of lesbian women, and that cervical abnormalities are found in women who do not have sex with men.[10,11] In addition, or because of this, human papillomavirus vaccination rates are low in SMW.[12,13]

Rates for mammography screening are less consistent. Although some studies found lower rates of routine examinations in SMW when compared with heterosexual women,[8,9] others found fairly high rates of screening.[5,14,15] The lack of inclusion of sexual orientation/identity and behavior when gathering and presenting national statistics for breast cancer makes it difficult to know the actual prevalence in lesbians. There is evidence of increased rates of known risk factors for breast cancer in SMW, such as increased body mass, high alcohol intake, and nulliparity in lesbians compared with heterosexual women.[16–21]

Research has demonstrated that SMW reported most types of vaginitis, but gonorrhea, herpes, and syphilis were reported only by women who also had sex with men.[22,23] A careful sexual history is necessary to determine risk because SMW often report a history of past male partners, sometimes within the last year.[24] Bacterial vaginosis is commonly found in lesbians and their female partners, and can be spread between female partners.[25] Rates of human immunodeficiency virus infection are generally low, but higher in SMW who have sex with high-risk men, use intravenous or other drugs, and/or are sex workers.[26] Researchers suggest an increased emphasize should be placed on the need for history taking related to sexual partners and drug use among women who have sex with women. This measure can better assess risk, and may open the discussion about prevention of human immunodeficiency virus and other sexually transmitted infections.

Care of Sexual Minority Women in Childbirth and Parenting

Increasingly, SMW are having children through donor insemination and adoption. Areas of potential concern for care are (1) finding a sensitive birthing provider and a sensitive, inclusive place for the birth, (2) worry about coming out to the provider and hospital staff, (3) decisions about donors and drafting legal agreements, (4) involvement of the nonpregnant female partner, (5) legal issues between partners regarding the child, and (6) extended family support for the pregnancy and child.[3]

First, SMW who wish to become pregnant may have to select and then come out to a provider. In addition, decisions about whether to use a known or unknown donor, how much interaction to have with the donor, and how much to tell the child about their conception must be made.[27] The Human Rights Campaign has written materials to help make these decisions[28] (http://www.hrc.org). Unfortunately, written materials focused on heterosexuals and that use terms such as "husband or male partner" do not make SMW feel welcome or included. Partners may not feel welcome in prenatal groups, the delivery room, and hospital environments, which are set up for heterosexual couples.[2] The partner has no legal relationship to the child unless the couple is married or have completed a second parent adoption agreement. The pregnant woman needs to anticipate and ask if her partner will be able to participate in the birthing process.[29]

A recent study found 3 major themes of stress in same-sex parenting that they thought might represent unique risk factors for perinatal depression. Those themes include (a) disappointment over lack of family support, (b) difficulty negotiating parenting roles, and (c) legal and political barriers.[30] Children of lesbian parents have challenges owing to social stigma, but studies found these children are comparable with children raised in heterosexual families in relation to their social and psychological adjustment and development.[31–33] Physical and sexual abuse was found less frequently in these families,[32] and children were found to be less constrained by gender roles.[34]

SPECIFIC RISK FACTORS AND HEALTH CARE PROBLEMS OF SEXUAL MINORITY WOMEN

Most research involving SMW demonstrates a generally healthy population and without increased rate of medical diagnoses (except asthma), such as cardiovascular disease, hypertension, diabetes mellitus, arthritis, pulmonary disease, and cancer. Risk factors related to medical diseases such as obesity, increased tobacco and alcohol use, psychological distress, and increased mental health disorders have been reported. Increased childhood sexual abuse (CSA) and intimate partner violence are also reported.[7–26,35–39]

Obesity and Overweight

Overweight and obesity are consistently found in the SMW population. A metaanalysis of early surveys of lesbians found a significantly higher prevalence of obesity, and they were less likely to consider themselves to be overweight.[8] A newer review of the literature on high body mass index (BMI) in lesbians found that these women were more likely to be overweight or obese, and to be more accepting of it.[40] Lesbians in a more recent analysis of the Nurses Health Study II reported increased BMIs (compared with heterosexual women).[41] Community studies also found that lesbians had higher BMIs than heterosexual women.[20,42–44] In addition, analyses of data from national[45] and state[36,46] surveys, as well as national college health surveys,[47] confirmed that SMW had a higher prevalence of overweight and obesity than all other female sexual orientation groups across age groups and throughout the United States.[14]

Overweight and obesity in SMW are associated with older age, poorer health status, lower educational attainment, relationship cohabitation, and lower exercise frequency.[21,48] Explanations for higher BMIs posit that SMW are less concerned about weight because they are not socialized to adhere to traditional standards of appearance,[40] and they find women with higher BMIs to be more attractive.[49,50] Attitudes toward weight may vary with age, and younger SMW are more concerned about their weight than older lesbians.[51] Several studies found a relationship between CSA and higher rates of obesity in SMW.[42,43,52]

Few data exist on interventions to reduce weight in lesbians. SMW are interested in programs related to weight loss, but are more motivated by becoming healthy and fit rather than by being thin.[51] Lesbians may favor having lesbian-only groups for weight loss so they feel comfortable discussing their lives and may be more comfortable bringing partners when appropriate and helpful.[51] A key variable in working with SMW is tailoring weight management programs to the needs, goals, and community norms of SMW.[53,54]

Tobacco Use

Cigarette smoking is more common among SMW.[8,55,56] Data from state surveys in California demonstrated smoking rates among lesbian and bisexual women to be about10% to 12% higher than among heterosexuals.[57] Data from the Nurses' Health Study II also found that lesbians had a greater risk of tobacco use during adolescence, which was mediated by childhood abuse.[58] Childhood physical abuse was related to earlier age of smoking onset, as well as current smoking status.[59]

Alcohol Use and Abuse

Early studies of SMW found high rates of alcohol use; in some studies, it was almost 5 times that of heterosexual women. More recent studies, with improved sampling and methodology, continue to show higher rates of use and abuse in SMW when compared with heterosexual women. Women who report same sex sexual partners use alcohol more frequently, in greater amounts, and report greater alcohol-related morbidity than women with opposite sex partners.[60,61] About 1 in every 5 SMW (18%), compared with 2% of heterosexual women, report having been in alcohol recovery.[62] In a California Health Maintenance Organization, SMW were more likely to drink and drink heavily, independent of the effects of stress, depression, and socioeconomic variables.[63] Nationally representative data from the National Epidemiologic Survey of Alcohol and Related Conditions found that 60% of SMW met the criteria for substance use disorder, compared with 24% of heterosexual women.[64] Bisexual women have the highest rates of alcohol use and abuse,[65] and alcohol abuse may also be related to a history of CSA.[62,66,67]

Mental Health Problems

Higher rates of depression and mental health problems exist in SMW.[17,68–70] It is posited that stigma and the stress of being a minority may be related to the high rate of depression.[71] Stress related to being a sexual minority, feeling stigmatized, internalized homophobia, and lack of social support have been related to low self-esteem, psychological distress, and depression.[72–75] Recent studies dividing SMW into lesbian and bisexual groups found more complex results. One study analyzed National Epidemiologic Survey of Alcohol and Related Conditions data and reported that women with only women partners had a lower number of mood disorders when compared with bisexual women. The highest percentage of mood disorder (58.7%) was found among bisexual women, whereas 44.4% was reported by the lesbian sample, 36.5% in the "not sure about sexual identity," and 30.5% in the heterosexual group.[76]

Childhood Sexual Abuse

CSA may be found in more than twice as many SMW as heterosexuals.[77] A review of the literature found that SMW have lifetime sexual assault rates ranging from 16% to 85% and the median estimate was 30%. This rate is strikingly higher than the range of 11% to 17% for women in general.[78] Data from the National Study of Health and Life Experiences of Women found that CSA was more prevalent among lesbians than heterosexuals, was more severe, and was more likely to be perpetrated by a male relative.[79,80] Bisexual women reported the highest rates of CSA, with the longest duration, and highest rates of physical force.[80]

CSA, a frequent finding among women who report adverse childhood events, is associated with multiple negative chronic health conditions in adults.[81] Despite overwhelming evidence to support a relationship between adverse childhood events and health among adults, few primary care providers have translated the need for collecting these data or knowledge about treatment into practice.[82,83]

Smoking, high alcohol use and abuse, depression and anxiety, and obesity have been discussed as related to CSA in SMW. This information is important when working with SMW in any context, but especially when working with abuse and sexual issues. Screening for CSA and exploring the relationship between these issues and abuse may be crucial to treating depression and anxiety, decreasing tobacco and alcohol use, and weight control. Researchers suggest that eating disorders, tobacco use, and excessive alcohol use may serve as self-nurturing strategies to relieve depression and anxiety, or to decrease the stress seen among survivors of CSA.[62] Being overweight may shield survivors of CSA from feeling or being overtly sexual, and this factor may decrease anxiety.

RECOMMENDATIONS FOR THE HEALTH CARE OF SEXUAL MINORITY WOMEN

Based on research findings, several recommendations for health care of SMW can be made. Even though lesbians are becoming more comfortable in health care settings and are coming out to health care providers in greater numbers, providers can increase comfort by being welcoming in a variety of ways. Lesbians feel more included if health questionnaires and educational materials are use gender-neutral language, and are inclusive via language such as using partner instead of husband. Similarly, educational materials that are not gender specific are more culturally sensitive and allow SMW to feel accepted and included.

Asking all patients, "Do you have sexual attractions or sexual relationships with men, women, both, or neither?" provides the opportunity for women to disclose their sexual preferences and sexuality. If the woman discloses that she is having sex with another woman, ascertain if she has disclosed this to her social network, and discuss how comfortable she is in telling her family, friends, coworkers, and other health care providers about her sexuality and her lifestyle. Many SMW are anxious in social settings, and hide or lie about their partners and their life style, which can cause anxiety and depression. An understanding of available resources and referrals for SMW who are not forthcoming about their sexuality can assistance them during the coming out process. Similarly, SMW may find it difficult to know who will be welcoming and knowledgeable when choosing a health care provider, and advertisement in gay media or making an explicit reference to welcoming SMW in promotional materials is useful.

Rates of physical examination and pap smears have increased over the past 20 years, yet SMW still do not have pap smears and do not receive human papillomavirus vaccine at the suggested rates. Heterosexual women receive routine screening and health maintenance as a part of the visit to obtain birth control, but SMW may not receive this same care because of the lack of need for birth control. SMW women need to know that they are still at risk for cervical cancer and should be encouraged to seek preventative services. The rate of breast cancer in lesbians (as opposed to heterosexual women) is not known, but there are increased risk factors among lesbians. SMW seem to be aware of their risk for breast cancer, and report frequent mammograms, but still need to be encouraged to comply with guidelines for screening.

A careful sexual history is useful in determining risks for sexually transmitted infections, because many women who identify as SMW may have had or currently have male partners. Although chlamydia, gonorrhea, and syphilis are not frequently identified in women who have sex with women, bacterial vaginosis is common and can be transmitted from woman to woman. Human immunodeficiency virus is uncommon in lesbians, but may be found in women who use intravenous drugs, have sex with high-risk men, or are commercial sex workers, irrespective of their sexual identity.

SMW may report different norms related to body weight and appearance, and this calls for a different approach to healthy lifestyle and treatment recommendations. SMW may need weight reduction interventions specifically related to increasing their health and fitness rather than tailored to fitting the societal norm for female appearance or matching a "normal BMI." Discussions about the importance of their body type to the woman, as well as her partner, are crucial to effect change. Clinicians need to be aware of treatment options for SMW in their communities to assure comfort in discussing their everyday lives and involving the partner in the process.

Mental health problems, especially anxiety and depression, are common among SMW and have an effect on weight status, as well as the rates of smoking, and alcohol use and abuse. The stigma of being an SMW, stresses of disclosure/nondisclosure, and lack of social support are keys in the development and continuance of "minority stress." Assessing for a history of mental health problems and screening for current mental health symptoms, along with any indicated referrals to mental health providers who are SMW sensitive, are critical elements in caring for SMW. Screening for tobacco and alcohol use and referral to treatment is also especially necessary. Mental health and addiction services are critical to the care of other health problems in this population because psychosocial concerns have a negative effect on general health.

The relationship of obesity to CSA in SMW raises issues in health care treatment. Although there is evidence of higher rates of sexual abuse in SMW and the relationship of CSA to other health issues, there are few recommendations in the literature related to how to intervene. Asking about a history of CSA and exploring how it has affected their health is especially necessary when working with SMW. Little evidence exists regarding the mechanisms between CSA and smoking, mental health problems, alcohol abuse, and obesity, thus, making it difficult to reliably predict their presence in any woman.

SUMMARY

SMW are common in all health care settings, but may be invisible to providers unless practitioners ask every patient about sexual attractions, behaviors, and identity. Written and promotional materials welcoming SMW and written in gender-neutral language are essential. Screening for cancers and sexually transmitted infections must be done according to published protocols. No medical conditions are significantly more commonly found in SMW, but diagnoses such as overweight/obesity, tobacco and alcohol abuse, mental health problems, and a history of CSA are common and are risk factors for other diseases. These factors intertwine when treating each of the problems. SMW need to be able to comfortably come out and express their concerns. Methods for working on those concerns in the health care environment must be explored.

REFERENCES

1. Institute of Medicine. The health of lesbian, gay, bisexual and transgender people: building a foundation for better understanding. Washington, DC: National Academies Press; 2011.
2. Buchholz S. Experiences of lesbian couples during childbirth. Nurs Outlook 2000; 48:307–11.
3. McManus AJ, Hunter LP, Renn H. Lesbian experiences and needs during childbirth: guidance for healthcare providers. J Obstet Gynecol Neonatal Nurs 2006; 35:13–23.
4. Klitzman RL, Greenberg JD. Patterns of communication between gay and lesbian patients and their health care providers. J Homosex 2000;42:65–75.
5. Roberts SJ, Patsdaughter CA, Grindel C, et al. Health related behaviors and cancer screening of lesbians: results of the Boston Lesbian Health Project II. Women Health 2004;39:41–55.

6. Haider AH, Schneider EB, Kodadek LM, et al. Emergency department query for patient-centered approaches to sexual orientation and gender identity: the EQUALITY study. JAMA Intern Med 2017;177(6):819–28. Available at: http://jamanetwork.com/pdfaccess. ashx?url=/data/journals/intemed/0/on 4/24/2017.

7. Matthews AK, Hughes TL, Osterman GP, et al. Complementary medicine practices in a community based sample of lesbians and heterosexual women. Health Care Women Int 2005;26:430–47.

8. Cochran SD, Mays VM, Bowen D, et al. Cancer-related risk indicators and preventive screening behaviors among lesbian and bisexual women. Am J Public Health 2001;91:591–7.

9. Powers D, Bowen DJ, White J. The influence of sexual orientation on health behaviors in women. J of Prevent & Intervent in the Community 2001;22:4–60.

10. Agenor M, Krieger N, Austin SB, et al. Sexual orientation disparities in Papanicolaou test use among US women: the role of sexual and reproductive health services. Am J Public Health 2014;104:e68–73.

11. Matthews AK, Brandenburg DL, Johnson TP, et al. Correlates of underutilization of gynecological cancer screening among lesbian and heterosexual women. Prev Med 2004;38:105–13.

12. Marazzo JM, Koutsky LA, Kiviat NB, et al. Papanicolaou test screening and prevalence of genital human papillomavirus among women who have sex with women. Am J Public Health 2001;91:947–52.

13. McRae AL, Katz ML, Paskett ED, et al. HPV vaccination among lesbian and bisexual women: findings from a national survey of young adults. Vaccine 2014;32(37):4736–42.

14. Aaron DJ, Markovic N, Danielson ME, et al. Behavioral risk factors for disease and preventive health practices among lesbians. Am J Public Health 2001;91:972–5.

15. Burnett CB, Steakley CS, Slack R, et al. Patterns of breast cancer screening among lesbians at increased risk for breast cancer. Women Health 1999;29:35–55.

16. Brandenburg DL, Matthews AK, Johnson TP, et al. Breast cancer risk and screening: a comparison of lesbian and heterosexual women. Women Health 2007;45(4):109–30.

17. Case P, Austin SB, Hunter DJ, et al. Sexual orientation, health risk factors, and physical functioning in the Nurses' Health Study II. J Womens Health 2004;13:1033–47.

18. Diamant AL, Wold C. Sexual orientation and variation in physical and mental health status among women. J Womens Health 2003;12:4–49.

19. Dibble S, Roberts SA, Nussey B. Comparing breast cancer risk between lesbians and their heterosexual sisters. Womens Health Issues 2004;14:60–8.

20. Roberts SA, Dibble SL, Nussey B, et al. Cardiovascular risk in lesbian women. Womens Health Issues 2003;13:167–74.

21. Yancey AK, Cochran SD, Corliss HL, et al. Correlates of overweight and obesity among lesbian and bisexual women. Prev Med 2003;36:676–83.

22. Roberts SJ, Sorensen L, Patsdaughter C, et al. Sexual behaviors and sexually transmitted diseases of lesbians: results of the Boston Lesbian Health Project. J Lesbian Stud 2000;4:49–70.

23. Bauer GR, Welles SL. Beyond assumptions of negligible risk: sexually transmitted diseases and women who have sex with women. Am J Public Health 2001;91:1282–6.

24. Marrazzo JM, Stine K. Reproductive health history of lesbians: implications for care. Am J Obstet Gynecol 2004;190:1298–304.
25. Marrazzo JM, Koutsky LA, Eschenbach DA, et al. Characterization of vaginal flora and bacterial vaginosis in women who have sex with women. J Infect Dis 2002; 185:1307–13.
26. Mays VM, Cochran SD, Pies C, et al. The risk of HIV infection for lesbians and other women who have sex with women: implications for HIV research, prevention, policy and services. Women's Health: Research on Gender, Behavior and Policy 1996;2:119–39.
27. Haimes E, Weiner K. " Everybodys got a dad … " Issues for lesbian families in the management of donor insemination. Sociol Health Illn 2000;22:477–99.
28. Human Rights Campaign Donor Insemination: the basics. Available at: http://www.hrc.org/resources/donor-insemination-the -basics. Accessed June 13, 2017.
29. Harvey SM, Carr C, Bernheine S. Lesbian mothers: health care experiences. J Nurse Midwifery 1989;34:115–9.
30. Ross LE, Steele L, Sapiro B. Perceptions of predisposing and protective factors for perinatal depression in same-sex parents. J Midwifery Womens Health 2005; 50:65–70.
31. Bos HMW, van Balen F, van den Boom DC. Lesbian families and family functioning: an overview. Patient Educ Couns 2004;59:263–75.
32. Gartrell N, Rodas C, Deck A, et al. The national lesbian family study: interviews with the 10-year-old children. Am J Orthopsychiatry 2005;75:518–24.
33. Golombok S, Perry B, Burston A, et al. Children with lesbian parents: a community study. Dev Psychol 2013;9:20–33.
34. Stacey J, Biblarz TJ. How does the sexual orientation of parents matter? Am Sociol Rev 2001;66:159–83.
35. Caceres BA, Brody A, Luscombe RE, et al. Systematic review of cardiovascular disease in sexual minorities. Am J Public Health 2017;107(4):e13–21.
36. Conron K, Mimiaga MJ, Landers S. A population based study of sexual orientation identity and gender differences in adult health. Am J Public Health 2010; 100(10):1953–60.
37. Eliason M. Chronic physical health problems in sexual minority women: review of the literature. LGBT Health 2014;1(4):259–68.
38. Frederiksen-Goldsen KL, Hyun-Jun K, Barkan SE, et al. Health disparities among lesbian, gay, and bisexual adults: results from a population-based study. Am J Public Health 2013;103(10):1802–9.
39. Gonzales G, Przedworski BS, Henning-Smith C. Comparison of health and health risk factors between lesbian, gay and bisexual adults and heterosexual adults in the United States. JAMA Intern Med 2016;176(9):1344–51.
40. Bowen DJ, Balsam KF, Ender SR. A review of obesity issues in sexual minority women. Obesity (Silver Spring) 2008;16(2):221–8.
41. Jun J, Corliss HL, Nichols LP, et al. Adult body mass index trajectories and sexual orientation. The nurses health study II. Am J Prev Med 2013;42(4):348–54.
42. Smith HA, Markovic N, Danielson ME, et al. Sexual abuse, sexual orientation and obesity in women. J Womens Health 2010;19(8):1–8.
43. Smith HA, Markovic N, Hughes T. Sexual abuse, sexual orientation and obesity in women. J Womens Health 2010;19(8):1525–32.
44. Zaritsky E, Dibble SL. Risk factors for reproductive and breast cancers among older lesbians. J Womens Health 2010;19(1):125–31.

45. Boehmer U, Bowen DL, Bauer G. Overweight and obesity in sexual-minority women: evidence from population-based data. Am J Public Health 2007;97(6): 1134–40.

46. Deputy NP, Boehmer U. Weight status and sexual orientation: differences by age and within racial and ethnic subgroups. Am J Public Health 2014;104(5):103–8.

47. Struble CB, Lindley LL, Montgomery K, et al. Overweight and obesity in lesbian and bisexual college women. J Am Coll Health Assoc 2010;59(1):51–6.

48. Brittain DR, Dinger MK, Hutchinson SR. Sociodemographic and lesbian-specific factors associated with physical activity among adult lesbians. Womens Health Issues 2013;23(2):e103–8.

49. Cohen AB, Tannenbaum IJ. Lesbian and bisexual women's judgements of the attractiveness of different body types. J Sex Res 2004;38(3):226–32.

50. Swami V, Tovee MJ. The influence of body mass on the physical attractiveness preferences of feminist and nonfeminist heterosexual women and lesbians. Psychol Women Q 2006;30:252–7.

51. Roberts SJ, Stuart-Shor E, Oppenheimer R. Lesbians' attitudes and beliefs regarding overweight and weight reduction. J Clin Nurs 2010;19:1986–94.

52. Aaron D, Hughes T. Association of childhood sexual abuse with obesity in a community sample of lesbians. Obesity (Silver Spring) 2007;15(4):1023–8.

53. Garbers S, McDonnall C, Fogel SC, et al. Aging, weight and health among adult lesbian and bisexual women: a meta synthesis of the multisite "Healthy Weight Initiative" focus groups. LGBT Health 2015;2(2):176–87.

54. Haynes S. Healthy weight: a new tailored approach for lesbian and bisexual women. Womens Health Issues 2016;26(Suppl 1):S4–6.

55. Hughes TL, Jacobson KM. Sexual orientation and women's smoking. Curr Womens Health Rep 2003;3(3):254–61.

56. Cochran SD, Bandiera FC, Mays VM. Sexual orientation-related differences in tobacco use and second hand spoke exposure among US adults aged 20-59: 2003-2010 National Health and Nutrition Examination Surveys. Am J Public Health 2013;103(10):1837–44.

57. Gruskin EP, Greenwood GL, Matevia M, et al. Disparities in smoking between the lesbian, gay and bisexual population and the general population in California. Am J Public Health 2007;97(8):1496–502.

58. Jun H, Austin SB, Wylie SA, et al. The mediating effect of childhood abuse in sexual orientation disparities in tobacco and alcohol use during adolescence: results from the Nurses Health Study II. Cancer Causes Control 2010;21(11):1817–28.

59. Matthews AK, Cho YI, Hughes TL, et al. The influence of childhood physical abuse on adult health status in sexual minority women: the mediating role of smoking. Womens Health Issues 2013;23(2):e95–102.

60. Cochran SD, Keenan C, Schober C, et al. Estimates of alcohol use and clinical treatment needs among homosexually active men and women in the U.S. population. J Consult Clin Psychol 2000;68(6):1062–71.

61. Cochran SD, Mays VM. Relation between psychiatric syndromes and behaviorally defined sexual orientation in a sample of the US population. Am J Epidemiol 2000;151(5):516–23.

62. Hughes TL, Johnson T, Wilsnack SC. Sexual assault and alcohol abuse: a comparison of lesbians and heterosexual women. J Subst Abuse 2001;13(4):515–32.

63. Gruskin EP, Hart S, Gordon N, et al. Patterns of cigarette smoking and alcohol use among lesbians and bisexual women enrolled in a large HMO. Am J Public Health 2001;91:976–9.

64. McCabe SE, Hughes TL, Bostwick WB, et al. Sexual orientation, substance use behaviors and substance dependence in the US. Addiction 2009;104: 1333–43.

65. Burgard SA, Cochran SD, Mays VM. Alcohol and tobacco use patterns among heterosexually and homosexually experienced California women. Drug Alcohol Depend 2005;77:61–70.

66. Wilsnack SC, Hughes TL, Johnson TP, et al. Drinking and drinking-related problems among heterosexual and sexual minority women. J Stud Alcohol Drugs 2008;69:129–39.

67. Roberts SJ, Grindel C, DeMarco R, et al. Lesbian use and abuse of alcohol: results of the Boston Lesbian Health Study II. Subst Abus 2004;25(4):1–9.

68. Razzano LA, Cook JA, Hamilton MM, et al. Predictors of mental health services use among lesbian and heterosexual women. Psychiatr Rehabil J 2006;29(4): 289–98.

69. Boehmer U, Maio X, Linkletter C, et al. Health conditions in younger, middle, and older ages: are there differences by sexual orientation? LGBT Health 2014;1(3): 168–76.

70. Matthews AK, Hughes TL, Johnson T, et al. Prediction of depressive distress in a community sample of women: the role of sexual orientation. Am J Public Health 2002;92(7):1131–9.

71. Meyer I. Prejudice, social stress, and mental health in lesbian, gay, and bisexual populations: conceptual issues and research evidence. Psychol Bull 2003; 129(5):674–97.

72. Lehavot K, Simoni JM. The impact of minority stress on mental health and substance use among sexual minority women. J Consult Clin Psychol 2011;79(2): 159–70.

73. Lewis RJ, Derlega VJ, Griffin JL, et al. Stressors for gay men and lesbians: life stress, gay-related stress, stigma consciousness, and depressive symptoms. J Soc Clin Psychol 2003;22(6):716–29.

74. Oetjen H, Rothblum ED. When lesbians aren't gay: factors affecting depression among lesbians. J Homosex 2000;39(1):49–73.

75. McGregor BA, Carver CS, Antoni MH, et al. Distress and internalized homophobia among lesbian women treated for early stage breast cancer. Psychol Women Q 2001;25:1–9.

76. Bostwick WB, Boyd C, Hughes TL, et al. Dimensions of sexual orientation and the prevalence of mood and anxiety disorders in the United States. Am J Public Health 2010;100(3):468–75.

77. Hughes TL, Szalacha LA, Johnson TP, et al. Sexual victimization and hazardous drinking among heterosexual and sexual minority women. Addict Behav 2010;35: 1152–6.

78. Rothman F, Exner D, Baughman AL. Systematic review of 75 studies that examine the prevalence of sexual assault victimization among gay or bisexual men and lesbian or bisexual women. Trauma Violence Abuse 2011;12(2):55–66.

79. Alvy LM, Hughes TL, Kristjanson AF, et al. Sexual identity group differences in child abuse and neglect. J Interpers Violence 2013;28(10):2088–111.

80. Wilsnack SC, Kristjanson AF, Hughes TL, et al. Characteristics of childhood sexual abuse in lesbians and heterosexual women. Child Abuse Negl 2012;36: 260–5.

81. Kalmakis KA, Chandler GE. Adverse childhood experiences: towards a clear conceptual meaning. J Adv Nurs 2014;70(7):1489–501.

82. Kalmakis K, Chandler G, Roberts SJ, et al. Nurse practitioner screening for childhood adversity among adult primary care patients: a mixed-method. J Am Assoc Nurse Pract 2017;29(1):35–45.

83. Gustafson TB, Sarwer DB. Childhood sexual abuse and obesity. Obes Rev 2004; 5:129–35.

High-Risk Pregnancy

Nola Holness, CNM, ARNP (Adult), MSN, PhD

KEYWORDS

- High-risk pregnancy • Risk assessment • Perception • Physical • Psychological
- Spiritual care

KEY POINTS

- Any condition associated with a pregnancy with an actual or potential hazard to the well-being of the mother or fetus is considered a high-risk pregnancy.
- The situations and conditions that create high-risk pregnancy status are varied.
- Careful risk assessment and individualized care are needed for each pregnancy.

A pregnant woman has the potential for risks during pregnancy, labor, and birth. Any unexpected or unanticipated medical or obstetric condition associated with pregnancy with an actual or potential hazard to the health or well-being of the mother or fetus is considered a high-risk pregnancy.[1–3] Worldwide, 20 million women have high-risk pregnancies and more than 800 die daily from perinatal conditions.[4,5] The percentages of high-risk pregnancies range from 6% to 33% because the situations and conditions that constitute high-risk pregnancy are varied.[3,6,7] Throughout the world, 5% to 10% of all pregnancies are complicated by preeclampsia.[8] Other pregnancy challenges are malaria, tuberculosis, and chronic iron deficiency anemia.[9] For women with high-risk pregnancies, the goal is adequate antenatal care, timely management and treatment, and expert care during labor, delivery, and postpartum to reduce maternal and infant mortality.[5]

INCIDENCE OF HIGH-RISK PREGNANCIES IN THE UNITED STATES

The Centers for Disease Control and Prevention (CDC)[10] report that 65,000 women in United States are affected annually by high-risk pregnancies with severe complications resulting in high medical, hospital, and rehabilitations costs. In the United States, the CDC[11] reported the incidence of 3 major high-risk conditions: hypertensive disorders, postpartum hemorrhage, and deep vein thrombosis (DVT). In 2012, hypertensives disorders occurred in 86 of every 1000 pregnancies. Between the years of 1994 and 2012, the incidence of postpartum hemorrhage quadrupled from 0.5 per

Disclosure Statement: No commercial or financial conflicts of interest or any funding sources.
Florida International University, 100 Luna Park Drive, Apartment #139, Alexandria, VA 22305, USA
E-mail address: nholness@fiu.edu

1000 to 2 per 1000 and pulmonary embolism, a complication of DVT, doubled from 0.1 per 1000 to 0.2 per 1000. Gestational diabetes occurred in 2% to 10% of all pregnancies in the United States in 2012.[8] In addition, the rates of multiple births increased from 19 per 1000 to 33 per 1000 births with many resulting in preterm infants. Pregnancies with preterm births cost $26 billion annually.[12] Thus, high-risk pregnancies continue to be a major medical dilemma in the United States.

CLASSIFICATION OF HIGH-RISK PREGNANCIES

The National Institutes of Health[8] has outlined several broad categories that may create risks during a pregnancy. These risks are outlined in **Table 1**. According to the CDC, there are specific indicators of severe maternal morbidity.[11] These indicators are listed in **Table 2**. Risks may also be classified as biophysical, psychosocial, sociodemographic, or environmental factors as expanded in **Table 3**. Other factors to assess when determining pregnancy risks are outlined in **Box 1**. These indicators are even more important for women from vulnerable populations.[13] Risk assessment is needed for these high-risk pregnancy situations.

RISK ASSESSMENT OF HIGH-RISK CONDITIONS

Screening in pregnancy is the standard of care to identify any condition that may negatively impact the mother or fetus.[14] At any point during pregnancy, challenges to maternal and fetal health may occur, including disorders before or at the beginning of the pregnancy, during pregnancy, or problems and conditions associated with labor, delivery, and the postpartum period.[9] Risk assessment is needed to determine when increased attention is needed.[9] A detailed history, thorough physical examination, and laboratory findings may reveal potential mortality or morbidity risks for the mother or fetus.[14,15(p633)]

PERINATAL OUTCOMES

Fetal and maternal pregnancy risks may result in poor perinatal outcomes. Kiely and colleagues[16] purported that sociodemographic and behavioral conditions may affect the perinatal health of the mother and fetus more than pregnancy-related situations. Those risks include obesity (body mass index [BMI] >31.9), smoking, employment status (full-time vs part-time), education attained (less than high school, high school/GED, or some college), intimate partner violence, and depression. In that study involving

Table 1 National Institutes of Health: high-risk pregnancy categories	
Existing health conditions	Hypertensive disorders, polycystic ovarian syndrome, diabetes, renal disease, autoimmune disease, thyroid disease, infertility, obesity, HIV/AIDS
Age	Adolescent First-time pregnancy after 35 y of age
Lifestyle factors	Alcohol use Tobacco use Illicit drug use
Conditions of pregnancy	Multiple gestation Gestational diabetes Preeclampsia and eclampsia

Abbreviation: HIV, human immunodeficiency virus.

Table 2
Centers for Disease Control and Prevention: severe maternal morbidity indicators

Cardiovascular	Acute myocardial infarction Cardiac arrest/ventricular fibrillation Disseminated intravascular coagulation Thrombotic embolism Blood transfusion Cardio monitoring Conversion of cardiac rhythm
Pulmonary	Adult respiratory distress syndrome Pulmonary edema Temporary tracheostomy Mechanical ventilation
Injuries	Intracranial injuries Internal injuries of thorax, abdomen, or pelvis
Pregnancy specific	Amniotic fluid embolism Eclampsia Puerperal cerebrovascular disorders
Operative	Severe anesthesia complications Hysterectomy Operations on heart and pericardium Cardiac arrest during procedure or surgery
Other	Acute renal failure Sepsis Shock Sickle cell anemia with crisis Aneurysm

African American women, perinatal outcomes related to low birth weight (birth weight of ≤2499 g at any gestational age), very low birth weight (birth weight ≤1500 g), preterm birth (before the completion of 37 weeks of pregnancy), cesarean delivery, miscarriage, neonatal intensive care unit (NICU) admission, and perinatal death were examined.[16] Education was the strongest predictor of preterm birth, whereas BMI was the strongest predictor of low birth weight, cesarean delivery, miscarriage, NICU admission, and perinatal death.[16]

The Behavioral Risk Factor Surveillance System found that 52% of women 18 to 44 years old reported at least one risk factor before pregnancy and 18% had at least 2 factors.[17] Risk factors included smoking, drinking, obesity, diabetes, and mental distress, with obesity as the most common risk (23%).[17] Yet, how a woman perceived her perinatal risk varies.

Table 3
General categories of high-risk pregnancy

Biological	Genetic, nutritional, general health status, medical, or obstetric disorders
Psychological	Maternal behaviors, lifestyle, emotional disorders, disturbed interpersonal relationships, inadequate social support, unsafe cultural practices
Sociodemographic	Lack prenatal care, insurance status, low income, marital status, race, ethnicity
Environmental	Hazards in workplace and general environment, chemicals, gases, radiation

---

Box 1
Determinants of pregnancy risks

1. Pregnancy intention, prenatal care initiation, barriers

2. Folic acid use, maternal drug, tobacco, and/or alcohol use

3. Preconception health, including family planning methods, maternal weight before pregnancy, most recent seasonal flu vaccine, oral health

4. Prepregnancy medical conditions, in particular hypertension and diabetes

5. Physical and emotional abuse, actual/potential stress, social support, depression

---

THE PREGNANT WOMAN'S PERCEPTION OF RISK

Risk perception is defined as "a person's expectancy about the probability of an event."[2(p416)] How a pregnant woman defines her risks may affect her willingness to seek obstetric care and follow prescribed regimens of care.[2]

In a study of nulliparous women, 5 factors affected how they viewed their risks in the pregnancy; pregnancy-related anxiety (most significant), medical risk (reproductive history, medical condition, complications of pregnancy), maternal age, gestational age, and perceived inner control.[2(p423)] Other factors that may affect a pregnant woman's risk perception are her social constructs and experiences, prior life experiences, influence of the health care provider (HCP), public information, previous situational experience, and her personal philosophy.[14,18] In general, a woman with a high-risk pregnancy may process the need for care of herself and her fetus relative to employment status, other children, partner, culture, family history, or past personal experiences.[1(p10)]

VARIATIONS IN PERCEPTIONS OF RISK DURING PREGNANCY

Identifying risk during pregnancy does not always indicate that a poor outcome will occur. Some pregnancies with risk factors result in a normal pregnancy, labor, and recovery, whereas those with no known risk factors develop problems.[14] Thus, it has been argued that there is no exact definition of risk in pregnancy, as risk may be perceived in different ways by the woman and by her HCP.[18] The pregnant woman sees a "potential for loss or damage," whereas her provider assesses risk as a "statistical calculation of odds and ratio."[18(p653)] The statistical aspect to risk assessment is based on how likely it is that the event will occur, whereas the psychological portion hinges on how the woman views her risk.[1] She may not view her risk as being as severe as the nurse does or as other HCPs view them.[1] In addition, HCPs may be influenced by concerns related to litigation.[13] The opinions of health care professionals and her individual circumstance, including socioeconomic status, as well as her own intuition may affect how she assesses the severity of risk.[1(p9)] Because she may not view her risk in similar ways as her HCP, problems may arise in communication; there may be lack of satisfaction and failure to use necessary health care resources[1(p10)] when the pregnancy is labeled as high risk.

THE HIGH-RISK PREGNANCY LABEL

Labeling a pregnancy as high risk may create varied responses. The woman may develop negative emotions, with feelings of vulnerability[3] and mental stress.[9,14] The high-risk label may lead to additional testing, which may be unnecessary and can result in a loss of the sense of control over the pregnancy. In addition, increased fear and anxiety regarding pregnancy and birth may develop.[14] The pregnant woman with a high-risk condition who develops birth fear may be influenced by the media, her family, and the medical community.[14(p196)] Some terms and statements she hears may be interpreted as serious and/or are complex, and this may further diminish her sense of control.[19] Conversely, the label of high risk may not affect some women negatively, as they view the HCP and technology in a positive light.[3(p139)] Risk assessment and care of the pregnant woman with actual or potential complications must, therefore, be evidenced based.[14]

PRENATAL PHYSICAL ASSESSMENT IN HIGH-RISK PREGNANCIES

For women with chronic medical conditions or risky health behaviors, care needs to start before pregnancy to improve preconception health.[16] Programs should seek to increase consumer knowledge and highlight the potential benefits of preconception counseling to reduce risk factors and negative outcomes.[13,16] Consideration of and screening for high-risk conditions during pregnancy are primary and secondary prevention strategies. For example, assessing for the current-season flu vaccine and providing that injection is primary prevention. Secondary prevention testing for a disease when a woman is asymptomatic helps to reduce the impact of that process.[14] Prenatal care, education, and counseling should be personalized and emotionally supportive, especially for a woman identified with a high-risk pregnancy.[6]

Ongoing monitoring of high-risk pregnancies is essential. Electronic fetal monitoring antenatally, especially in the third trimester, evaluates uteroplacental functioning to detect fetal well-being or compromise.[15(pp633–651)] **Table 4** outlines additional options for biophysical assessment of fetal well-being.[15] Biochemical assessments of maternal blood or amniotic fluid are also essential during a high-risk pregnancy. These assessments may be useful to identify fetal lung maturity, open neural tube defects, and genetic disorders.[15] **Table 5** provides information on common biochemical assessments.

PSYCHOLOGICAL IMPACT OF A HIGH-RISK PREGNANCY

Emotions play a significant part in a woman's response to her high-risk pregnancy. She may experience a contradictory mixture of emotions as seen in **Box 2**. Some

Table 4 Biophysical assessment of fetal well-being	
Daily fetal movement	Noninvasive, reassuring sign of fetal health, especially during third trimester; protocols for counting vary; in general 2–3 times daily, minimum of 10 movements in 12 h expected
Ultrasonography	Assesses fetal activity, gestational age, fetal growth, fetal and placenta anatomy, amniotic fluid volume, visualization for invasive tests
MRI	Evaluate fetal structure and growth, placenta, quantity of amniotic fluid, maternal structures
Nonstress test	External electronic monitoring of fetal heart rate response to movement, contractions, other stimulation
Modified biophysical profile	Combines nonstress test with measurement of quantity of amniotic fluid using ultrasound
Vibroacoustic stimulation	Combines sound and vibration to stimulate fetus
Contraction stress test	Stimulate uterine contractions to assess fetal response to stress

Table 5
Biochemical assessment of fetal well-being

Coombs test	First prenatal visit and when indicated; detects Rh and other antibodies in fetal blood that may cause fetal incompatibility with maternal antigens
Cell free DNA testing	10 wk; noninvasive screening for genetic disorders, fetal Rh status, sex, single gene disorders
Chorionic villus sampling	10–13 wk; transcervical or transabdominal to assess fetal tissue for genetic conditions
Multiple markers	11–14 wk screen for chromosomal and other abnormalities; maternal sero-markers include pregnancy-associated placental protein, hCG, ADAM 12, inhibin A; ultrasound markers include fetal nuchal translucency, fetal nasal bone. Second-trimester screening markers include MSAFP, unconjugated estriol, hCG
Amniocentesis	After 14 wk; transabdominally to obtain amniotic fluid with fetal cells to assessment genetic disorders, neural tube defects, pulmonary maturity, hemolytic disease
Alpha fetoprotein	15–20 wk; screen for neural tube defects via MSAFP, or diagnostic via amniotic fluid alpha fetoprotein measurement
Percutaneous umbilical blood sampling	Second and third trimester; invasive, to access fetal circulation for fetal blood sampling and transfusion

Abbreviations: ADAM 12, disintegrin and metalloproteinase 12; hCG, human chorionic gonadotropin; MSAFP, maternal serum alfa fetal protein.

broad themes include the desire to have a child, acknowledging the existing health problem, overcoming the initial shock of a newborn with health problems, and coping with the intense feelings associated with having a sick newborn while experiencing frustrations, desires, and surmounting problems associated with the pregnancy.[4(pp1189–1193)] The psychological stress experienced during a high-risk pregnancy may result from multiple events. These events may include family separation (if hospitalized) and communication with professionals. Other stressors are the environment, health status of the mother and baby, self-image, emotions, family status,[12(p398)] informational support, self-esteem, age, and depression.[20] In a qualitative study of women with severe maternal morbidity, they described their experiences as being difficult, painful, and suffering and noted a fear of losing the child. However, some were able

Box 2
Emotional responses to a high-risk pregnancy

1. Joy of being pregnant[19]
2. Fear (uncertainty of the unknown, lack of information about high-risk pregnancy)
3. Anxiety (anxiety related to potential interruption of the pleasantness of pregnancy)
4. Sorrow (loss of a baby during a previous pregnancy, lack of planning, and negative situations associated with a high-risk pregnancy)[19(p3)]
5. Happiness (overcoming problems, related to support received)[19]
6. Frustration, anger, hope[1]
7. Shock, depression, guilt, loneliness, mood swings[12(p404)]

to look ahead to overcoming the negative experience, surviving the care, and taking the baby home.[4]

High-risk pregnancies result in higher postpartum depression rates (9%–12%) when compared with women with low-risk pregnancies.[7] Contributing factors include maternal age, gravidity, number of abortions, interval between pregnancies, and the desirability of pregnancy.[7(p107)] Although postpartum depression is common, in women with high-risk pregnancies, emotions of "guilt, inadequacy, and uneasiness" may result in higher levels of depression.[21(p2)] Disbelief and denial may also be experienced.[6]

When trying to understand reasons for pregnancy complications, coping with internal conflicts, and in searching for the meaning of the experience, women may to turn to faith.[12] Spirituality is a deeply personal determinant of health, which may give meaning to women with high-risk pregnancies.[22] In a small study, women admitted for high-risk pregnancy conditions tried to connect with what was sacred to them. For these women, the high-risk pregnancy was associated with increased feelings of guilt, despair, and hopelessness. Staying spiritually connected helped them cope with negative emotions. They reported a sense of restored hope and more positive feelings.[22(p64)] Although they admitted to struggling with spiritual beliefs during crises (such as a high risk pregnancy), faith, religious traditions, and their relationship with their God or spiritual realm provided them with increased calmness and strength to cope.[22(p67)]

NURSING IMPLICATIONS FOR HIGH-RISK PREGNANCIES

Optimal care for a high-risk pregnancy may avert a negative impact on the mother and fetus and can result in positive outcomes and reduced adverse outcomes.[13,14] Nurses can foster an environment of security and trust during preconception, antenatal, intrapartal, and postnatal care, which will enhance the health and well-being of the mother and fetus.[4] Medical and nursing care of women with high-risk diagnoses must be specific. Maternal diabetes care includes blood sugar monitoring and possible insulin use. In addition, preterm labor management requires uterine activity monitoring, fluids, medication, and limited physical activity. Hypertension care is focused on medication and stress relief.[23(p179)]

Challenges to effective care for high-risk conditions include adherence to medical treatments, overall health, reduction of risk behaviors, and attending early and frequent prenatal care.[23(pp178–179)] Pregnant women with high-risk conditions face many prenatal (physiologic and health related) and postpartum challenges (physiologic and psychosocial). Environmental challenges of residence, sanitation, and income may also have a compounded effect on health and well-being.[23]

It is important to identify complications, develop protocols, and provide care.[24] Thus, the World Health Organization's Sustainable Development Goals and the Global Strategy for Women's, Children's and Adolescents' Health states an objective to reduce the global maternal mortality ratio.[5] In 2015, the maternal mortality ratio was 239 per 100,000 live births in developing countries and 12 per 100,000 live births in developed countries.[5] Key strategies to meet the goal of reducing the maternal mortality ratio to less than 70 per 100,000 live births are listed in **Box 3**. At the national level, strategies targeting low-income minority groups must alleviate disparity in diseases burden and access to care, reduce risk behaviors, and improve health outcomes.[25] In addition to conditions of national and global concerns, such as depression, human immunodeficiency virus, and malaria,[9] other essential national maternal and infant health indicators to assess effectiveness of policies and programs must be resolved (**Box 4**).[25(pp2495)] As maternal morbidity rates continue to increase in

---

Box 3
Global strategies to reduce maternal mortality

1. Increase research and evidence-based clinical and programmatic guidance through high-quality data collection to assess needs and identify priorities for care.

2. Set global standards for and accountability of member states to ensure universal health coverage for comprehensive reproductive, maternal, and newborn health care.

3. Provide technical support to member states to strengthen health systems.

4. Advocate for more affordable and effective treatments; design training materials and guidelines for health workers to address inequalities in access to quality reproductive, maternal, and newborn health care services.

5. Support countries to implement policies and programs and monitor progress.[5]

---

the United States, a national initiative, Alliance for Innovation on Maternal Health, seeks to reduce maternal morbidity/mortality through multidisciplinary collaboration of state and health system teams using evidenced-based established protocols to improve maternal outcomes for women, including those with high-risk pregnancies.[26]

Nurses have multiple roles when caring for women with high-risk specialized, yet individualized needs.[27] Nurses become managers of coordinated care, teachers and counselors in encouraging healthy behaviors, and promoters of active participation in shared decision-making.[27(pp478–479)] A motivated nurse must convey the importance of prenatal care.[27] The high rates of maternal and fetal morbidity and mortality should prompt nursing actions to monitor women and reduce adverse outcomes. Some nursing strategies to care for clients with high-risk pregnancies include[27(p479)] home or clinic consult visits by nurses, lay visitors, or advanced practice nurses[23] and periodic telephone calls by advanced practice nurses to support and monitor high-risk clients.[23,27] Other helpful approaches would be to identify and strengthen the woman's support systems and to evaluate her emotional and physical state as well as that of her partner.[27] Fetal movement monitoring by the client is an appropriate action with which the client can partner with her providers in ongoing assessment of her high-risk pregnancy.[27]

Maternal fetal medicine physicians, highly skilled nurses (including advanced practice nurses, such as nurse midwives, women's health, and neonatal nurse

---

Box 4
National maternal and infant health indicators

1. Previous low birth weight

2. Previous preterm birth

3. Gestational diabetes or other diabetes

4. Hypertension during pregnancy

5. Placenta previa, placenta abruption

6. Urinary tract or kidney infection

7. Preterm labor

8. Preterm premature rupture of fetal membranes

9. Infant admitted to NICU

practitioners), NICU staff, social workers, nutritionists, and all who interact with the mother and family during a high-risk pregnancy should provide an interprofessional approach to create as positive an environment as possible.[1,27,28] Through collaboration of shared expertise, physicians and advanced practice nurses can enhance the health of the mother and fetus by comanaging complex care.[23] Collaboration and communication is a powerful determinant of reduced mortality for women with high-risk pregnancies.[23(p179)]

HOSPITALIZATION

Women with complicated pregnancies may require lifestyle changes, medication regimens, technical support, and even hospitalization.[3(p137)] Depending on the condition, some women with high-risk situations may require hospitalization for weeks or months before the baby's birth. Physical changes that may result from being hospitalized on bed rest include muscle atrophy, cardiovascular deconditioning, and bone loss.[3,12]

In the antepartum setting, the hospitalized woman may experience increased fear, loss of control, powerlessness, loneliness, anger, and anxiety.[3(pp139),12] To improve her psychological status, nursing interventions could revolve around celebrating milestones, such as significant gestational ages, for example, 28 or 32 weeks. Other approaches to addressing psychological factors include planning a special meal for her and her family, assisting her to verbalize her fears, and providing support from others, including mental health counselors, family counselors, neonatal educators.[12(p406)] Modified visiting hours, informational support, and group therapy for hospitalized high risk pregnant women may provide beneficial emotional support to reduce feelings of isolation and depression.[20]

EMOTIONAL AND SPIRITUAL CARE

Communication of risk is important; but how communication occurs may influence decisions, as heightened fear and anxiety may be the response. When HCPs are aware of these emotions, they can focus on helping alleviate negative feelings by creating a trusting environment, keeping her informed of her gestational status, and facilitating her participation in decisions about care.[1,14,19]

In addition, nurses who care for high-risk pregnant women encounter their own stressful situations with uncertainties regarding the status of mother and fetus, and the outcome of the pregnancy. It is key that nurses do not label women as negligent or irresponsible but must try to see and understand each woman's individual circumstance.[1(p12)] Nurses and other HCPs need to be aware of personal communication styles when interacting with pregnant women[1] and may need training courses to address communication skills, such as use of open-ended questions and verbal cues, when addressing the biopsychosocial needs of women with high-risk pregnancies.[7]

All care should be of high quality, with individualized communication tailored to the woman's needs; but emotional and spiritual care are especially enhanced by therapeutic communication. Another component of care is the spiritual health of women with high risk pregnancies. An empathetic environment allowing for prayer, meditation, and other practices of value to the woman are means by which HCPs can enhance spiritual well-being.[21] For example, relaxation techniques may reduce depression. Women in an experimental group were given a relaxation protocol conducted in a passive peaceful environment. The women, in comfortable positions, were given a mental exercise, sat quietly, did deep breathing exercises, targeted muscle relaxation, and said the number *one* quietly to themselves for 10 to 20 minutes.[22] They were advised to take a mental trip to somewhere they enjoyed or would enjoy visiting. When finished they sat quietly for a few more minutes before standing.[22(p3)] The control group had usual care. Both groups had similar depression scores at admission. Five days later, the intervention group reported less depression.[22] Prenatal and postnatal nurses could use this strategy to reduce depression and anxiety.

SUMMARY

The joy of being pregnant may be dimmed by the diagnosis of an existing or potential high-risk condition for the mother and/or fetus. One woman with a high-risk pregnancy may not view her condition as serious or life threatening, whereas another may be emotionally overcome by such a diagnosis. The situations and conditions that create a high-risk status are varied; thus, careful risk assessment and individualized care are needed for each pregnancy.[18,23,28] Despite a high-risk pregnancy, which may carry the potential for severe maternal or fetal harm, most pregnant women have great expectations for a positive outcome. Collaborative physical, emotional, cultural, and spiritual care and support is needed from multiple health care personnel to promote the wellness of the mother and fetus.

REFERENCES

1. Lee S. Risk perception in women with high-risk pregnancies. Br J Midwifery 2014; 22(1):8–13.
2. Bayrampour H, Heaman M, Duncan KA, et al. Predictors of perception of pregnancy risk among nulliparous women. J Obstet Gynecol Neonatal Nurs 2013; 42(4):416–27.
3. Rodrigues PB, Zambaldi CF, Cantilino A, et al. Special features of high-risk pregnancies as factors in development of mental distress: a review. Trends Psychiatry Psychother 2016;38(3):136–40.
4. Carvalheira AP, Tonete VL, Parada CM. Feelings and perceptions of women in the pregnancy-puerperal cycle who survived severe maternal morbidity. Rev Lat Am Enfermagem 2010;18(6):1187–94.
5. World Health Organization. Maternal mortality. 2016. Available at: http://www.who.int/mediacentre/factsheets/fs348/en/. Accessed April 29, 2017.
6. Poplar J. Holistic care in high risk pregnancy. Int J Childbirth Educ 2014;29(4): 68–71.
7. Zadeh MA, Khajehei M, Sharif F, et al. High-risk pregnancy: effects on postpartum depression and anxiety. Br J Midwifery 2012;20(2):104–13.
8. Eunice Kennedy Shriver National Institute of Child Health and Human Development. What are the factors that put a pregnancy at risk?. Available at: https://www.nichd.nih.gov/health/topics/high-risk/conditioninfo/pages/factors.aspx. Accessed April 29, 2017.
9. Queenan JT, Spong CY, Lockwood CJ, editors. Index, in protocols for high-risk pregnancies: as evidence-based approach. Chichester (United Kingdom): John Wiley& Sons, Ltd; 2015. https://doi.org/10.1002/9781119001256.index.
10. Centers for Disease Control. Data on selected pregnancy complications in the United States. 2016. Available at: https://www.cdc.gov/reproductivehealth/maternalinfanthealth/pregnancy-complications-data.htm. Accessed April 29, 2017.
11. Centers for Disease Control. Severe maternal morbidity in the United States. 2016. Available at: https://www.cdc.gov/reproductivehealth/maternalinfanthealth/severematernalmorbidity.html. Accessed April 30, 2017.

12. Rubarth LB, Schoening AM, Cosimano A, et al. Women's experience of hospitalized bed rest during high-risk pregnancy. J Obstet Gynecol Neonatal Nurs 2012; 41(3):398–407.
13. Ahluwalia IB, Harrison L, Simpson P, et al. Pregnancy risk assessment monitoring system and the W.K. Kellogg Foundation joint project to enhance maternal and child health surveillance: focus on collaboration. J Womens Health 2015;24(4):257–60.
14. Jordan RG, Murphy PA. Risk assessment and risk distortion: finding the balance. J Midwifery Women's Health 2009;54(3):191–200.
15. Lowdermilk D, Perry S, Cashion K, et al. Maternity and women's health care. 11th edition. St Louis (MO): Elsevier; 2016.
16. Kiely M, El-Mohandes AA, Gantz MG, et al. Understanding the association of biomedical, psychosocial and behavioral risks with adverse pregnancy outcomes among African-Americans in Washington DC. Matern Child Health J 2011;15:S85–95.
17. Denny CH, Floyd RL, Green PP, et al. Racial and ethnic disparities in preconception risk factors and preconception care. J Womens Health 2012;21(7):720–9.
18. Carolan MC. Towards understanding the concept of risk for pregnant women: some nursing and midwifery implications. J Clin Nurs 2009;18(5):652–8.
19. Wilhelm LA, Alves CN, Demori CC, et al. Feelings of women who experienced a high-risk pregnancy: a descriptive study. Online Braz J Nurs 2015;14(3):1–6. Available at: http//www.scielo.br/scielo.php?pid=S0034-7167201100016&script=sci arttext. Accessed March 7, 2017.
20. Denis A, Michaux P, Callahan S. Factors implicated in moderating the risk for depression and anxiety in high risk pregnancy. J Reprod Infant Psychol 2012; 30(2):124–34.
21. Price S, Lake M, Breen G, et al. The spiritual experience of high-risk pregnancy. J Obstet Gynecol Neonatal Nurs 2007;36(1):63–70.
22. Araujo WS, Romero WG, Zandonade E, et al. Effects of relaxation on depression levels in women with high-risk pregnancies: a randomized clinical trial. Rev Lat Am Enfermagem 2016;24:e2806.
23. Brooten D, Youngblut J, Blais K, et al. APN-physician collaboration in caring for women with high-risk pregnancies. J Nurs Scholarsh 2005;37(2):178–84.
24. Azevedo RO, Silvino ZR, Ferreira HC. Nursing guidelines with regard to high-risk pregnancy: a descriptive study. Online Braz J Nurs 2013;12(Suppl):623–5. Available at: http://www.objnursing.uff.br/index.php/nursing/article/view/4512. Accessed March 7, 2017.
25. Dietz P, Bombard J, Mulready-Ward C, et al. Validation of self-reported maternal and infant health indicators in the Pregnancy Risk Assessment Monitoring System. Matern Child Health J 2014;18:2489–98.
26. Council on Patient Safety in Women's Health Care. About AIM. Available at: http://safehealthcareforeverywoman.org/aim-program/about-aim/. Accessed January 4, 2018.
27. Rodrigues ARM, Rodrigues DP, Viana AB, et al. Nursing care in high-risk pregnancies: an integrative review. Online Braz J Nurs 2016;15(3):472–84. Available at: http://www.objnursing.uff.br/index.php/nursing/article/view/5434. Accessed March 7, 2017.
28. Brooten D, Youngblut JM, Donahue D, et al. Women with high-risk pregnancies, problems, and APN interventions. J Nurs Scholarsh 2007;39(4):349–57.

Helping Mothers Reach Personal Breastfeeding Goals

Diane L. Spatz, PhD, RN-BC

KEYWORDS

• Human milk • Anticipatory guidance • Anatomy • Physiology

KEY POINTS

- In order for families to make an informed infant feeding decision it is essential that they are fully educated on the science of human milk and breastfeeding.
- Starting breastfeeding requires time and commitment, and it is not always easy or natural.
- Mothers should seek help immediately if they run into breastfeeding challenges.
- Peer and professional support are essential for a mother to reach her personal breastfeeding goals.

INTRODUCTION

Professional organizations worldwide recommend exclusive human milk/breastfeeding for the first 6 months of life, and continued breastfeeding with appropriate complementary foods for 1 year or more.[1–3] Despite the growing interest in breastfeeding and although more than 80% of women in the United States initiate breastfeeding, exclusivity and breastfeeding continuation rates remain suboptimal.[4] A mere 22% of infants are exclusively breastfed for the first 6 months and only 31% of infants are breastfed for one full year.[4]

There are also racial/ethnic and economic disparities. Breastfeeding initiation rates in white women are 84.3% compared with only 66.3% of black women. Women in the lowest poverty ratio have breastfeeding initiation rates of only 66.3%, whereas women in the highest poverty ratio have initiation rates of 91.7%. Additionally, enrollment in the Women Infant and Children (WIC) program seems to have a negative influence on breastfeeding, with women who are not WIC eligible having breastfeeding initiation rates of 91.1%. Women who are not in WIC but eligible have initiation rates of 82% and women enrolled in the WIC program have the lowest rates of initiation at only 74.1%.[4]

The author reports no conflict of interest related to this article.
Department of Family and Community Health, The University of Pennsylvania School of Nursing, The Children's Hospital of Philadelphia, 418 Curie Boulevard, Philadelphia, PA 19104, USA
E-mail address: spatz@nursing.upenn.edu

Nurs Clin N Am 53 (2018) 253–261
https://doi.org/10.1016/j.cnur.2018.01.011
0029-6465/18/© 2018 Elsevier Inc. All rights reserved.

The WIC program spends 25 times more money on the purchase of infant formula as compared with the provision of breastfeeding support.[5] Clearly there is much work to be done to improve mothers' ability to reach personal breastfeeding goals.

The Centers for Disease Control and Prevention have identified nine key strategic areas with sufficient research evidence as topics to focus on to improve the landscape of breastfeeding in the United States[6]

- Improving maternity care practices to support breastfeeding mothers
- Increasing health care providers education and knowledge
- Ensuring mothers have access to professional lactation assistance
- Peer-to-peer support for breastfeeding mothers
- Workplace support for breastfeeding mothers
- Support for breastfeeding in early care and education
- Access to breastfeeding education and information
- Social marketing
- Addressing the marketing of infant formula

This article focuses on the importance of prenatal messaging and goal setting to ensure that mothers are able to optimize their milk supply during the critical window of opportunity in the first 2 weeks after delivery. This focus was chosen because national research data from the Infant Feeding Practices data set found that the largest categories of why women stopped breastfeeding were for reasons related to milk supply, or concerns that the infant was not getting enough nutrition or gaining enough weight.[7]

At the Children's Hospital of Philadelphia, where the author practices, all mothers receive a personalized one-to-one prenatal lactation consultation during the second or third trimester. This is focused on the science of human milk, the physiology of lactation, and the importance of prenatal goal setting. Our clinical practice and research demonstrate that this approach is effective at achieving not only high breastfeeding initiation rates (99%) but also high exclusive human milk rates (54% at 3 months; 35% at 6 months) and longer breastfeeding duration (median, 8 months) despite some mothers having infants who were critically ill at birth and spent time in a neonatal intensive care unit.[8]

THE SCIENCE OF HUMAN MILK

For families to make an informed infant feeding decision it is essential that they are fully educated on the science of human milk and breastfeeding. It is not enough for families to know that breastfeeding is good, they must understand the dose-dependent nature of human milk and breastfeeding on health outcomes. **Table 1** depicts critical teaching areas related to the health benefits of human milk for all infants (including those who may start their life requiring intensive care).

In addition to reduced mortality and morbidities infants who are fed human milk have enhanced brain development and improved developmental outcomes. This has been demonstrated in term and preterm infants. Preterm infants who were human milk fed during the neonatal intensive care unit stay had increased white matter, brain size, and higher IQ.[13]

In infants born at less than 30 weeks of gestation when infants were fed more than 50% of enteral feeds from human milk, they had greater deep nuclear gray matter volume at the term equivalent age, better performance on IQ at age 7, greater academic achievement, better working memory, and better motor function.[14]

Similar findings have been noted in healthy-term breastfed infants. Deoni and colleagues[15] found that infants who were breastfed had significantly more white matter

Table 1
Human milk and breastfeeding risk reduction

Condition	Risk Reduction
Infant mortality	823,000 deaths annually[9] 13.6% vs 17.2% formula exposed for NICU infants[10]
Sudden infant death	36% for any breastfeeding longer than 1 mo[2]
Necrotizing enterocolitis	77% for NICU stay[2] 6.9% vs 16.7% (formula)[10]
Sepsis	19% vs 30.3% (formula)[10]
Otitis media	23% (any breastfeeding) 50% (3–6 mo)[2]
Lower and upper respiratory tract infections	63%–77% with exclusive breastfeeding >4–6 mo[2]
RSV	74% with breastfeeding >4 mo[2]
Improved feed tolerance and decreased number of days of TPN	NICU stay[11]
Retinopathy of prematurity	5.2% vs 9% (formula)[10]
Bronchopulmonary disease	47.7% vs 56.3% (formula)[10]
Asthma	26%–40% with breastfeeding >3 mo[2]
Leukemia	15%–20% with breastfeeding >6 mo[2]
Obesity	24% with any breastfeeding[2,12]
Type 1 and type 2 diabetes	30%–40%[2,12]
Long-term protection of gastrointestinal system (inflammatory bowel disease, Crohn's and celiac disease)	Any breastfeeding/>2 mo[2,12]

Abbreviations: NICU, neonatal intensive care unit; RSV, respiratory syncytial virus; TPN, total parenteral nutrition.

and scored higher on intelligence tests and had better developmental outcomes. Furthermore, research using functional MRI demonstrated that breastfed infants had more gray matter and better regional gray matter function.[16] Eight year olds who were breastfed as infants scored better on language and perception tasks.[16]

ANTICIPATORY GUIDANCE AND GOAL SETTING

Once families make an informed decision to breastfeed or provide human milk to their infant, it is important to provide appropriate anticipatory guidance and realistic expectations. Many women express fears and concerns regarding their ability to "successfully" breastfeed and when a mother runs into difficulties, it is common to hear the woman say "I feel like a failure." I have recently published a column regarding the importance of avoiding the word success with breastfeeding and instead, work with the mother and her family to set short-term, mid-term, and long-term breastfeeding goals.[17] Starting breastfeeding requires time, commitment, and it is not always easy or natural. Mothers and families should understand that it is important to make the investment in breastfeeding and seek help if they run into challenges.[17]

Mothers should be provided with appropriate and realistic expectations regarding the first few weeks of breastfeeding. At Children's Hospital of Philadelphia our message to the mother that her only job for the first 2 weeks after delivery is to eat, sleep, pump, and visit her baby. For a mother who has a healthy infant, her only job should be to eat, sleep, and breastfeed. Before delivery, the mother's family (however, she defines it), should be empowered to assume all other household responsibilities so that she can focus on feeding and making milk for her baby. It is essential for the mother and her family to understand that there is a critical window of opportunity following birth, and if she does not turn on all the prolactin receptor sites in her breasts and establish a normal milk supply early-on, she will not be a long-term breastfeeding mother.

Li and colleagues[7] study on why mothers stop breastfeeding in the first year of life found that after milk supply concerns, another major category of why mothers stop breastfeeding was a category related to "lactational factors" including such factors as pain, latch-on difficulties, nipple trauma, and discomfort. Kent and colleagues[18] reported that more than one-third (36%) of women seek help for persistent nipple pain, and that the most common cause of nipple pain (90%) was incorrect position and attachment.

When providing prenatal anticipatory guidance, it is important to teach mothers about the difference between pressure and pain. Mothers will and should feel pressure, because infants apply significant vacuum to the breast for milk removal. However, if a mother reports consistent and repetitive pain, this must be evaluated. Mothers should be advised that pain resolves for most women by an average of 18 days (range, 2–110 days).[18]

It is essential for mothers to understand the physiology of milk production and normal milk supply before delivery because this is a major reason that mothers stop breastfeeding. The breast begins to secrete milk at 16 weeks gestation; therefore, no matter how early a mother may deliver, she already has milk in her breasts and she is ready to fulfill all her infant's needs.

Additional anticipatory guidance for the family should address the mother's plan for return to work or school, and assisting her with a plan that allows a combination of breastfeeding and employment. The US Breastfeeding Committee provides excellence guidance on the Affordable Care Act and the law (See www.usbreastfeeding.org). Whereas some mothers may be able to access a free breast pump from their insurance, not all women are covered.

During the antenatal period, the mother and her family should order the pump either through their insurance or determine an option for pump rental or purchase if the mother will need to be away from her infant. Access to the highest quality breast pump assists the mother in being able to establish and maintain her milk supply long-term. It is critical to understand that if a mother is completely pump-dependent (no direct breastfeeding either because of infant hospitalization or maternal choice to pump and feed expressed milk), a hospital-grade breast pump is warranted.[19] The cost of feeding an infant formula for 1 year is estimated to be $1000 to $3000. The family should be educated that the cost of purchasing formula for one full year for their infant is significantly more than the cost of a one year pump rental or purchase of a personal use pump.

If the mother does plan to return to work, she should speak to her employer before her maternity leave and discuss options for breastfeeding or pumping once she returns to work. The Affordable Care Act only provides legal protection for mothers who have hourly paid employment. Women who are in salaried positions are not covered by the law. The Office of Women's Health provides workplace and space solutions for setting up pumping accommodations in a variety of work settings (refer to: https://www.womenshealth.gov/breastfeeding/employer-solutions/index.html).

Before delivery, the mother and her family should be provided with a resource list for breastfeeding services and peer-to-peer support. This could include World Wide

Web–based resources, telephone hotlines, and in-person peer or professional sup-port. The following is a listing of national World Wide Web–based resources that pro-vide evidence-based breastfeeding and lactation information.

- Centers for Disease Control and Prevention https://www.cdc.gov/breastfeeding/
- It's Only Natural Campaign (focused on African American families) https://www.womenshealth.gov/itsonlynatural/
- Human Milk Banking Association of North America https://www.hmbana.org/
- National WIC Association https://www.nwica.org/topics/breastfeeding
- The Office of Women's Health https://www.womenshealth.gov/breastfeeding/
- United States Breastfeeding Committee http://www.usbreastfeeding.org/

THE BIRTH HOSPITAL STAY FOR HEALTHY INFANTS

The Baby Friendly Hospital Initiative (BFHI) was developed to protect and support breastfeeding during the birth hospital stay.[20] There are 10 steps focused on improving breastfeeding practices for newborns immediately following birth:

- Step 1: Maintain a written breastfeeding policy that is routinely communicated to all health care staff
- Step 2: Train all health care staff in skills necessary to implement this policy
- Step 3: Inform all pregnant women about the benefits and management of breastfeeding
- Step 4: Help mothers initiate breastfeeding within 1 hour of birth
- Step 5: Show mothers how to breastfeed and how to maintain lactation, even if they are separated from their infants
- Step 6: Give infants no food or drink other than breast milk, unless medically indicated
- Step 7: Practice "rooming in," allow mothers and infants to remain together 24 hours a day
- Step 8: Encourage unrestricted breastfeeding
- Step 9: Give no pacifiers or artificial nipples to breastfeeding infants
- Step 10: Foster the establishment of breastfeeding support groups and refer mothers to them on discharge from the hospital or clinic

A 2017 publication from the World Health Organization (WHO) demonstrated that in 168 countries, only 10% of hospitals achieved this designation.[1] The BFHI guidelines were established 25 years ago; however, the 2017 WHO publication reported that despite the 25-year history no consistent improvement in breastfeeding outcomes was found globally.[1] Therefore, families should be aware that despite a hospital having achieved BFHI accreditation, there are questionable data about the effectiveness of the designation. Despite this the mother and her family should understand each of the 10 steps and develop a plan with health care professionals during the birth hospital stay to optimize her breastfeeding opportunities and experience.

FOR INFANTS REQUIRING INTENSIVE CARE

The BFHI does not specifically address the needs of critically ill or hospitalized infants (preterm, low birthweight, surgical) and the WHO recommends that vulner-able infants should be fed mother's own milk.[21] If an infant requires hospitalization, the Spatz 10 Steps for the Protection and Promotion of Human Milk and Breastfeed-ing in Vulnerable Infants serve as an evidence-based pathway with proven outcomes[22–24]:

- Step 1: Informed decision
- Step 2: Establishment and maintenance of milk supply
- Step 3: Human milk management
- Step 4: Oral care and feeding of human milk
- Step 5: Skin-to-skin contact
- Step 6: Nonnutritive sucking at the breast
- Step 7: Transition to direct breastfeeding
- Step 8: Measurement of milk transfer
- Step 9: Preparation for discharge
- Step 10: Appropriate follow-up

ESTABLISHMENT OF MILK SUPPLY AND "NORMAL" BREASTFEEDING

Following delivery of the placenta, the levels of estrogen, progesterone, and human placental lactogen rapidly decline signaling the mother's brain that the infant has arrived and this triggers the onset of the physiologic establishment of milk supply. For the mother to convert from lactogenesis I (colostrum) to lactogenesis II, frequent breast stimulation and emptying is essential.[25]

Mothers should be encouraged to hold their infants skin to skin as many hours of the day as feasible. Skin to skin contact is associated with improve breastfeeding outcomes for term and preterm infants. Mothers should be encouraged to breastfeed following the infants feeding cues; about every 1 to 3 hours. Frequent breast stimulation and emptying is essential to ensure the establishment of a full milk supply. Normal milk production is 440 to 1220 mL per a 24-hour period, with an average of 700 to 800 per day.[26]

During the first sixth months of exclusive breastfeeding, infants usually breastfeed in the following patterns[26]:

- Average 11 times at breast/day
- Range 6 to 19 times at breast/day
- Average time spent feeding is 2 hours and 18 minutes
- Only 14% had paired feeds (meaning the infant fed from both breasts at one feed)
- Average intake per feed = 76 g $\pm$ 40 g
- All infants <9 weeks fed at night
- Only 34% of infant >9 weeks did not feed at night (2200–0400)

If the infant is unable to directly breastfeed (ie, feed from the breast) the mother should be advised about the following principles of milk expression:

- Pump within 1 hour of delivery for earlier lactogenesis II and increased milk supply at 3 weeks postdelivery.
- Express milk with a hospital-grade electric pump every 2 to 3 hours, with a goal of eight or more pumping sessions per 24 hours.
- Continue to pump for at least 2 minutes after no milk flow is observed. Mothers have an average of 5.0 $\pm$ 2.0 milk ejections during pumping sessions and 62% of available milk is expressed during the first two milk ejections.[27]

Risk factors for delay in lactogenesis II include the following:

- Primigravida
- Obesity
- Pregnancy-induced hypertension and treatment with magnesium sulfate
- Gestational diabetes
- Antenatal steroids when delivery occurs 3 to 9 days following administration

- Polycystic ovarian syndrome (possibly)
- Influence of labor and delivery and breastfeeding support in the immediate post-partum period (amount of intravenous fluids during labor and delivery, the possible influence of exogenous oxytocin, ability to breastfeed or pump within the first hour after birth)

Conditions that may result in a mother being unable to establish a full milk supply include glandular hypoplasia (also known as insufficient glandular tissue of the breast), breast-reduction surgery, and breast augmentation surgery (depending on type). In instances when mothers are unable to establish a normal milk supply, the health care professional should provide support and counseling. Any amount of human milk is better than not receiving any mother's own milk. Mothers should be provided with scientific, evidence-based information regarding risk factors for the delay in lactogenesis II and conditions that may negatively impact the establishment of a full milk supply. It is critical that mothers be commended for their efforts at providing milk for their infant even if they cannot provide 100% of the infant's needs.

EFFECTIVE BREASTFEEDING

It is essential for the health professional to assess the ability of the infant to effectively breastfeed and transfer milk from the breast. Research demonstrates that vacuum is essential for milk removal.[28] To establish a full milk supply, the breasts must be effectively stimulated and emptied. If the infant is unable to latch and suckle effectively, the mother must be counseled to immediately start expressing milk by pumping so that her milk supply is not comprised.

NEONATAL WEIGHT LOSS AND APPROPRIATE SUPPLEMENTATION

The most important indication that breastfeeding is going well during the immediate postdelivery period is that the infant is having frequent meconium stools. Every time the infant breastfeeds effectively, the colostrum has a laxative effect and clears the bowel of the meconium. Urine output is not a good indicator of breastfeeding effectiveness in the immediate newborn period because most infants in the United States are born with a large exposure to maternal intravenous fluid during labor and delivery. Noel-Weiss and colleagues[29] found that at 72 hours there was a positive correlation between grams of weight lost and all maternal fluids ($P = .007$). Additionally, Chantry and colleagues[30] found that excessive fluid exposure was associated with excessive infant weight loss.

If supplementation is recommended, the mother should supplement in the smallest volume possible as recommended by the Academy of Breastfeeding Medicine Clinical Protocol on Appropriate Supplementation.[31] In the event a mother is instructed to supplement feeding, pumping with a hospital-grade electric breast pump is essential so that she can effectively convert from lactogenesis I to lactogenesis II.[19] It is imperative to understand that the first 2 weeks are critical for the establishment of milk supply. As health care providers this must be our first priority to ensure that mothers reach their personal breastfeeding goals.

SUMMARY

It is critical for health care providers to ensure that all women make an informed infant feeding choice. Breastfeeding is not a lifestyle choice but a public health issue.[2] Mothers need appropriate anticipatory guidance and support to achieve their personal breastfeeding goals.

REFERENCES

1. World Health Organization. Health topics: breastfeeding. 2017. Available at: http://www.who.int/topics/breastfeeding/en/. Accessed December 3, 2017.
2. American Academy of Pediatrics Work Group on Breastfeeding. Breastfeeding and the use of human milk. Pediatrics 2012;129(3):e827–41.
3. Association of Women's Health, Obstetric, and Neonatal Nurses. Breastfeeding. J Obstet Gynecol Neonatal Nurs 2015;44:145–50.
4. Centers for Disease Control and Prevention. Breastfeeding among U.S. children born 2002 – 2015. Available at: https://www.cdc.gov/breastfeeding/data/nis_data/index.htm. Accessed November 11, 2017.
5. Baumgartel K, Spatz DL, American Academy of Nursing Expert Breastfeeding Panel. WIC (special supplemental nutrition program for women, infants, and children): policy versus practice regarding breastfeeding. Nurs Outlook 2013;61(6): 466–70.
6. Centers for Disease Control and Prevention. Strategies to prevent obesity and other chronic diseases: the CDC guide to strategies to support breastfeeding mothers and babies. Atlanta (GA): U.S. Department of Health and Human Services; 2013. Available at: https://www.cdc.gov/breastfeeding/pdf/BF-Guide-508. PDF. Accessed November 11, 2017.
7. Li R, Fein SB, Chen J, et al. Why mothers stop breastfeeding: mothers' self-reported reasons for stopping during the first year. Pediatrics 2008;122:S69.
8. Martino K, Wagner M, Froh EB, et al. Post discharge breastfeeding outcomes of infants with complex anomalies that require surgery. J Obstet Gynecol Neonatal Nurs 2015;44(3):450–7.
9. Victora CG, Rollins NC, Murch S, et al. Breastfeeding in the 21st century. Lancet 2016;38:479–90.
10. Hair AB, Peluso AM, Hawthorne KM, et al. Beyond necrotizing enterocolitis prevention: improving outcomes with an exclusive human milk-based diet. Breastfeed Med 2016;11(2):70–4.
11. Ghandehari H, Lee ML, Rechtman DJ, H2MF Study Group. An exclusive human milk-based diet in extremely premature infants reduces the probability of remaining on total parenteral nutrition: a reanalysis of the data. BMC Res Notes 2012;5: 188.
12. Spatz DL, Lessen R. The risks of not breastfeeding-position statement. Morrisville (NC): The International Lactation Consultant Association; 2011.
13. Isaacs EB, Fischl B, Quinn BT, et al. Impact of breast milk on intelligence quotient, brain size, and white matter development. Pediatr Res 2010;67(4):357–62.
14. Belfort MB, Anderson PJ, Nowak VA, et al. Breast milk feeding, brain development, and neurocognitive outcomes: a 7-year longitudinal study in infants born at less than 30 weeks' gestation. J Pediatr 2016;177:133–9.e1.
15. Deoni SC, Dean DC, Piryatinsky I, et al. Breastfeeding and early white matter development: a cross-sectional study. Neuroimage 2013;82:77–86.
16. Ou X, Andres A, Pivik RT, et al. Voxel-based morphometry and fMRI revealed differences in brain gray matter in breastfed and milk formula-fed children. AJNR Am J Neuroradiol 2016;37(4):713–9.
17. Spatz DL. Say no to success-say yes to goal setting. MCN Am J Matern Child Nurs 2017;42(4):234.
18. Kent JC, Ashton E, Hardwick CM, et al. Nipple pain in breastfeeding mothers: incidence, causes and treatments. Int J Environ Res Public Health 2015;12(10): 12247–63.

19. Meier PP, Patel AL, Hoban R, et al. Which breast pump for which mother: an evidence-based approach to individualizing breast pump technology. J Perinatol 2016;36(7):493–9.
20. Baby Friendly USA. Available at: https://www.babyfriendlyusa.org/. Accessed December 3, 2017.
21. World Health Organization. Guidelines on optimal feeding of low birth-weight infants in low-and middle-income countries. 2011. Available at: http://www.who.int/maternal_child_adolescent/documents/9789241548366.pdf?ua=1.
22. American Academy of Nursing. 10 steps to promote and protect human milk and breastfeeding in vulnerable infants. 2015. Available at: http://www.aannet.org/initiatives/edge-runners/profiles/edge-runners-10-steps-to-promote-and-protect-human-milk. Accessed December 3, 2017.
23. Spatz DL. Ten steps for promoting and protecting breastfeeding in vulnerable populations. J Perinat Neonatal Nurs 2004;18(4):412–23.
24. Fugate K, Hernandez I, Ashmeade T, et al. Improving human milk and breast-feeding practices in the NICU. J Obstet Gynecol Neonatal Nurs 2015;44(3):426–38.
25. Wambach K, Riordan J. Breastfeeding and human lactation. 5th edition. Burlington (MA): Jones & Bartlett Learning; 2015.
26. Kent JC, Mitoulas LR, Cregan MD, et al. Volume and frequency of breastfeedings and fat content of breast milk throughout the day. Pediatrics 2006;117(3):e387–95.
27. Prime DK, Geddes DT, Hepworth AR, et al. Comparison of the patterns of milk ejection during repeated breast expression sessions in women. Breastfeed Med 2011;6(4):183–90.
28. Geddes DT, Kent JC, Mitoulas LR, et al. Tongue movement and intra-oral vacuum in breastfeeding infants. Early Hum Dev 2008;84(7):471–7.
29. Noel-Weiss J, Woodend AK, Peterson WE, et al. An observational study of associations among maternal fluids during parturition, neonatal output, and breastfed newborn weight loss. Int Breastfeed J 2011;6:9.
30. Chantry CJ, Nommsen-Rivers LA, Peerson JM, et al. Excess weight loss in first-born breastfed newborns relates to maternal lintrapartum fluid balance. Pediatrics 2011;127(1):e171–9.
31. Kellams A, Harrel C, Omage S, et al. ABM clinical protocol #3: supplementary feedings in the healthy term breastfed neonate, revised 2017. Breastfeed Med 2017;12:188–98.

Section IV: Older Adult

Menopause Symptom Management in the United Kingdom

Debra Holloway, RGN, MSc, FRCOG

KEYWORDS

- Menopause • Hormone replacement therapy (HRT)
- Premature ovarian insufficiency (POI) • Alternative therapies

KEY POINTS

- Menopause happens to all women as a midlife event with symptoms that vary.
- The views and research on hormone replacement therapy change, and nurses need to stay up to date because currently there may be fewer risks and more benefits.
- Hormone replacement treats most menopausal symptoms.
- Women with premature ovarian failure and hormone-dependent cancer need additional specialist care.
- Women with vaginal symptoms should be encouraged to use vaginal estrogens.

Menopause comes to all women. The timing and the severity of symptoms, however, are different in each woman. Linked to the type and severity of symptoms is the contact or lack thereof a woman may have with her health care provider. The world of menopause is confusing for women and for health care professionals alike. Often, published information contradicts a previous study, and it seems that only the negative findings get published within the popular press or women's magazines. It is hard for both women and health care professionals to stay current and be able to give balanced research-based advice.

The role of hormone replacement therapy (HRT) in the United Kingdom has changed completely over the past 10 to 20 years. In the 1980s, after menopause, most women were on HRT regimens. Subsequently, the publication of studies, such as the Women's Health Initiative[1] and Million Women Study[2] led to a decrease in HRT use by 70%.[3] Later reanalysis and the publication of the National Institute for Health and Care Excellence (NICE) guidelines[4] for the management of menopause established newer quality standards.[5] Currently, there is an increased interest in HRT and its role in the management of menopausal symptoms and in optimizing health at menopause and beyond.

No conflicts of interest.
Gynaecology, Guys and St Thomas NHS Foundation Trust, Mcnair Centre, Guys Hospital, Ground Floor Southwark Wing, London SE1 9RT, UK
E-mail address: Debra.Holloway@gstt.nhs.uk

Nurs Clin N Am 53 (2018) 263–277
https://doi.org/10.1016/j.cnur.2018.01.004   nursing.theclinics.com

The average age of menopause in the United Kingdom is 51 years old and has remained at this age for a long time. The range for a normal menopause is ages 45 to 55. Menopause is described as the cessation of the menstrual periods and is a retrospective event, confirmed when no menstruation has been noted for at least 1 year, unless there has been medically intervention to remove the ovaries.[4] This article discusses information related to women with a natural menopause. Women with special needs, such as premature ovarian insufficiency (POI), and women with induced menopause after cancer are discussed separately.

The period of time that leads up to the final menses is called perimenopause. It is characterized by fluctuations in hormone levels (luteinizing hormone [LH], follicle-stimulating hormone [FSH], and estradiol). Typically, the fluctuation of hormones produce irregular menstrual periods or changes in bleeding patterns as well as the classic menopausal symptoms of hot flushes/flashes (HFs), night sweats, mood changes, and poor sleeping.[4]

Globally, the age at which women have menopause has not changed over the past 100 years but the life expectancy has, and women now live 30 to 40 years or one-third of their life span in postmenopausal status.[6] Menopause should be a midlife event and is an excellent time to assess health needs in women to optimize their future health.

PATHOPHYSIOLOGY

Women are born with a finite number of oocytes, and these start to diminish in number as soon as a baby girl is born. When all the oocytes have been used, the ovaries are no longer responsive to FSH and LH. Those hormones are produced in a pulsatile pattern to stimulate the ovum to grow, develop, and be released. When the ovary does not respond to the feedback cycle, levels of FSH and LH rise and the production of estrogen by the ovary decreases.[6] The hormonal response of the ovary becomes erratic, leading to infrequent or more frequent periods before finally ending with amenorrhea. These changes also bring on symptoms in women that are classically believed complaints of menopause.[6] Until recently it was believed that HFs were related to low estrogen, but it has been shown that there is a more complex process that involves serotonin and noradrenaline.[6] That discussion is beyond the scope of this article. Research is under way, however, to look at genetics related to the ovary.[7] If a gene can switch off this process, it would give hope to many women who experience POI with no known cause.

SIGNS AND SYMPTOMS

A diagnosis of menopause does not require tests or investigations. In most women it is a diagnosis made related to symptoms and age.[4] Signs and symptoms vary among women. Some have none, others mild symptoms, and some severe cases, which leads to seeking help from medical professionals, alternative practitioners, or over-the-counter medication.

- Vasomotor—the most common and well-known symptoms are vasomotor symptoms (VMSs), HFs, and night sweats. These occur around perimenopause and into menopause. The amount, intensity, severity, and duration are unique to each woman. It was believed that HFs were short term, but in some cases they can be present for up to 20 years.[6] Although HFs are generally considered harmless, recent publications have shown a link with cardiovascular disease (CVD) and decreased bone density in women with persistent HFs.[8]
- Impaired sleep—linked with HFs, although sometimes a stand-alone complaint, is poor sleeping. Without a decent night's sleep, memory may become poor,

although this is also believed another sign of menopause. When not well rested, women can be confused and experience low mood, which can be mistaken for depression and poor self-esteem.[6]

- Bleeding—although not uncommon, irregular bleeding may warrant investigation. Depending on age of presentation, women with new intermenstrual bleeding or postcoital bleeding may need to be assessed for other diagnoses. Bleeding more than 1 year after the last menstrual period (LMP) (postmenopausal bleeding) and changes in bleeding patterns while on HRT are also reasons for additional testing, because postmenopausal bleeding can be a sign of endometrial, cervical, or vaginal/vulvar cancer.[4,6] Other causes of postmenopausal bleeding are listed in **Box 1**.

Abnormal bleeding needs to be investigated.[9] The first line of investigation for this is to take a history and perform a speculum examination, followed by an ultrasound scan. Then, depending on the endometrial thickness and any other pathology changes, a hysteroscopy should be performed. The endometrium thickness in postmenopausal women should be no more than 3 mm to 5 mm.[10] When the thickness is greater than 5 mm (depending on the guidelines in place), additional assessment is needed. There is currently some amount of debate, however, about the type and amount of further testing.[10] The thinner the endometrium, the more confident a practitioner can be that there is no pathology. In cases where it is thickened or there is significant bleeding, a hysteroscopy should be performed. This procedure normally is performed within the outpatient office and can be either diagnostic or operative.[11]

- Psychological symptoms—low mood, anxiety, irritability, mood changes, lack of energy, and fatigue may result from changes in hormones, and preexisting conditions can be made worse. Other events in a woman's life at this time can also have an impact on psychological symptoms. These might include caring for elderly parents, children leaving home, problems with a partner or job, and working life,[6] so history taking should include these factors as well.
- Libido changes—a woman's sex drive can be decreased from surgical and natural menopause. In addition to estrogen, the ovary secretes testosterone, which is important for libido and general well-being. This issue is a complex one, however, that does not correlate well with a reduction in testosterone. Other factors can include self-esteem and body image, poor sleep, anxiety, vaginal dryness, and pain with intercourse.[6]

Box 1
Causes of postmenopausal bleeding

- Vaginal atrophy
- Endometrial atrophy
- Endometrial pathology, such as polyps or fibroids
- Cervical pathology, such as cervical polyps
- Incorrect HRT/missing progestogen components of HRT
- Precancerous changes, such as hyperplasia
- Hormone-secreting ovarian tumors
- Endometrial cancer

- Urogenital symptoms—the bladder and the vagina have estrogen receptors and estrogen levels decreasing in menopause can affect both areas. Women may complain of vaginal dryness and vaginal pain. Vaginal dryness can lead to bleeding and pain when having sexual intercourse and in severe cases even bleeding from daily activities, such as walking. In some women, this may lead to avoidance of sexual intercourse due to pain, and libido may be affected as well.[6] In addition, women who are menopausal may not present for routine cervical screening due to pain and fear about the speculum examination.
Bladder symptoms include frequency, painful urination, and stress or urge incontinence. Women are reluctant and may need permission and encouragement to discuss these issues. They may even wait for a health care professional to bring vaginal and vulva problems up first.[12] One study of women with vulva and vaginal problems found that more than 40% had not discussed these issues with a health care professional.[12] Practitioners caring for women who are menopausal should have routine questions about urogenital symptoms to screen for distress and the need for interventions. Women may be too scared or embarrassed to discuss symptoms, such as dryness, burning, painful sex, prolapse, urgency, frequency, dysuria, and infections.[6]
- Other symptoms—the skin may become dryer, which causes itching. Some women may complain of bloating, joint pains, and weight gain.[4,6]
- A recent area that has been highlighted for women is menopause and work. The signs and symptoms, discussed previously, can all play a part in a woman's response to her workplace. Recently it has been recognized that menopausal women may need more help and accommodations for some workplace structures.[13,14]

CONTRACEPTION

Women around the time of perimenopause and menopause need advice related to contraception. Natural fertility declines, but women can still become pregnant.[15] Guidelines from the Faculty of Sexual and Reproductive Healthcare of the Royal College of Obstetricians and Gynaecologists[15] note the need to continue to use contraception for 2 years after the LMP when women are under 50 years of age and 1 year after the LMP if they are more than 50 years of age. There is no method of contraception that is absolutely contraindicated by age in the United Kingdom. As a woman gets older, however, she has higher risks of venous thromboembolism (VTE), CVD, and stroke.[15] Although this does not rule out the use of combined contraceptive pills, it does means that a careful history must be taken to assess for risk factors, such as overweight, obesity, and smoking. As alternatives, a progesterone-only pill can be used, or other methods of long-acting reversible contraception should be considered.[15] Depo-Provera (Pfizer Limited) (an injectable progesterone) should not be used in this age group due to its long-term effects on bone mineral density and bone loss. One useful type of contraceptive, the intrauterine system (IUS) provides long-term contraception and can decrease heavy menstrual bleeding or unpredictable bleeding.[15] HRT is not a contraceptive.

MENOPAUSE MANAGEMENT

Women who are menopausal should have their health optimized. The menopause is an ideal opportunity to give advice about lifestyle and diet to help combat weight changes and bone loss and possibly help with symptoms. Health and menopause advice can be either one-on-one, via groups, or via the Internet. Any information is beneficial to women around this time so they can increase their understanding of menopause and its symptoms and what help is available.

There are many approaches to resolving symptoms of menopause and there are mixed views as to whether simple strategies can help women with symptoms. The North American Menopause Society suggests that certain approaches may delay women from getting more effective treatment.[16] Women who cannot take or do not wish to take HRT or who have mild symptoms, however, may find some benefit in alternative treatments mainly for VMSs[17,18] (**Box 2**).

OVER-THE-COUNTER MENOPAUSE TREATMENTS/ALTERNATIVES

Some women may use other alternatives to prescribed medication or HRT if they are perceived to be natural and less harmful than taking medication. Some herbal medications, however, can have interactions with a prescribed medication, such as Sts John's wort. Some herbal products may also have an impact on underlying conditions, such as breast cancer, and there is little evidence and no well-controlled clinical trials on the impact they may have on symptoms and on overall health.[17]

There also can be issues with cost and the quality of the products. Some of the more popular alternatives are shown in **Box 3**.

Acupuncture for menopause symptoms has produced mixed results. Some studies suggest it may be beneficial, whereas others show no reduction in HFs but some improvement in quality of life and in sleep.[16,17]

Cognitive behavior therapy studies, mainly in women with breast cancer, reduced menopause symptoms and helped women cope with symptoms. Cognitive behavior therapy has been used in individual sessions, group sessions, by telephone, and as a self-guided activity.[17]

PRESCRIBED ALTERNATIVES

There are medications that can be prescribed to decrease VMSs and other symptoms of menopause. Unfortunately, there is a general lack of efficacy among these drugs. Due to that lack of efficacy from nonhormonal treatments, new areas are being looked

---

Box 2
Lifestyle advice actions and strategies that may help with menopausal symptoms

- Layer clothing and bed clothes
- Keep cool—facial spritz, fan, Chillow pillows
- Diet diary to look for any triggers, such as alcohol, caffeine, and spicy food
- Stop smoking (for health reasons alone),[6] and smokers have an earlier menopause[6] and more flushes[19]
- Reduce alcohol for health reasons, breast cancer risk, and bones[6]
- Weight loss[16]
- Relaxation
- Exercise for general health[16] (conflicting evidence in the role in VMSs)[18]
- Yoga/Pilates for general health and controlled breathing
- Increasing dietary input of plant estrogens (evidence limited)[16]

Box 3
Herbal alternatives for menopause symptoms

Red clover

Soy

Black cohosh

Yam

Maca

Hops

Dong quai

---

at. These include neurokinin B receptors, which look promising within small-scale studies.[20]

- Clonidine is the only licensed alternative in the United Kingdom and was originally used for the treatment of hypertension. In studies, it helps in approximately 30% to 40% of women[17] (bearing in mind a placebo effect from studies on HRT can be 30%–50%) and can cause side effects, such as dizziness, sleep problems, constipation, and hypotension.[6]
- Gabapentin can also be used for menopausal flushes[17] and may also help with joint pain, a menopause symptom and a side effect from aromatase inhibitors. It is not licensed, however, for this indication. When used, the starting dose is 300 mg, with increases to 900 mg as needed to control symptoms. Side effects include dizziness, weight gain, dry mouth, and unsteadiness.[16–18]
- Selective serotonin reuptake inhibitor/serotonin-norepinephrine reuptake inhibitors antidepressants, if used in lower doses, can help with VMSs.[16] NICE suggests that these should not be first-line treatments, because they are not as effective as HRT and do have side effects.[4] They do have a place, however, in women who cannot take estrogens. Examples that have evidence to suggest a reduction (although not licensed for this indication in the United Kingdom) are found in **Box 4**.

There may be some interaction with tamoxifen and fluoxetine or paroxetine along the cytochrome P450 pathway. One study found a risk of breast cancer recurrence in women taking paroxetine.[17] It was not clear, however, if it was a true drug interaction or if women were not taking the paroxetine because it was prescribed for depression and not for VMSs.[17] In general, venlafaxine may be safer to use with tamoxifen, and women have reported a reduction in HFs as well as better sleep.[21] The NICE guidelines state that

---

Box 4
Examples of selective serotonin reuptake inhibitors/serotonin-norepinephrine reuptake inhibitors

1. Paroxetine (10 mg)
2. Venlafaxine (37.5 mg–150 mg)
3. Escitalopram
4. Fluoxetine
5. Citalopram (10–30 mg)

---

antidepressants should not be a first-line treatment of women with menopausal symptoms because they are not as effective as HRT.[4] In addition, antidepressants have side effects, such as gastrointestinal disturbances, dry mouth, constipation, and reduced libido.[17] In general, the amount used for menopause symptoms is less than for depression; because of this, women can discontinue use without titrating down.

VAGINAL TREATMENT

The treatment of genitourinary symptoms during menopause is mainly estrogen.12 Women who cannot or do not want to use vaginal estrogens, however, can use vaginal moisturizers. All women should be encouraged to use vaginal lubrication when having intercourse if they are experiencing vaginal pain and dryness.

Depending on the problems a women experiences, treatment may just include vaginal estrogen. Women using systemic estrogens may find they do not need to use additional vaginal estrogens. Vaginal estrogens restore pH and thickened vaginal mucosa. Vaginal estrogens come as creams, pessaries, or vaginal rings. Creams are normally used nightly for 2 weeks, then twice a week as a long-term treatment. Unfortunately, when treatment is stopped, symptoms return. The NICE guidelines state indefinite use with no additional progesterone is safe, and there is no need for routine breaks or ultrasound scanning of the endometrium.[4]

There are few contraindications to vaginal preparations; however, the patient information leaflet may discourage use.[22] One contraindication is women taking aromatase inhibitors. Newer developments include ospemifene, a selective estrogen receptor modulator. This is delivered as a vaginal tablet. Unfortunately, the side effects are HFs and an increased risk of deep vein thrombosis. In addition, there are no safety data on women with breast cancer.[6]

Other options include vaginal bioadhesive moisturizers, such as Replens (LDS Consumer Products, Cedar Rapids, IA), and vaginal lubricants, such as Sylk (Freepost, Kingston upon Thames, England), which has a similar osmolarity and pH to vaginal secretions.[6,23] Vaginal laser therapy may help vaginal dryness by encouraging vaginal tissues to renew themselves. There are ongoing studies examining the role of laser therapy in treating bladder symptoms as well. There seem to be no side effects,[24] although long-term data are not available. The main drawback to its use in the National Health Service (NHS) in the United Kingdom is the cost of the laser.

HORMONE REPLACEMENT THERAPY

HRT is defined by its components and mode of delivery. The components are estrogen only versus estrogen and progestogen (combined) HRT. The modes of delivery are listed in **Table 1**.

Table 1 Hormone replacement therapy			
Type	Estrogen	Progestogen	Testosterone
Oral as tablet	Yes	Yes	No
Transdermal patch	Yes	Yes	No
Transdermal gel	Yes	Yes	Yes
Subdermal implant	Yes	No	Yes
Intrauterine	No	Yes	No
Vaginal	Yes	Yes (not licensed in UK)	Yes (not licensed in UK)

Women with a uterus need both estrogen (for the symptoms) and progesterone (to protect the endometrium from hyperplasia due to the effects of estrogen). There has been debate on the role of bioidentical hormones in HRT. The Food and Drug Administration and the British Menopause Society[25–27] have issued statements clearly stating the lack of evidence supporting claims that these compounded tailor-made preparations are better than standard preparations.[25]

When women are still perimenopausal and are having any periods, they need combined sequential HRT. This produces an endometrial shedding to prevent hyperplasia.[6] There are normally approximately 12 days to 14 days of progesterone per cycle.[3] If a woman does not want menstrual bleeding or is young, estrogen with an IUS can be used. Certain HRT regimes, called long cycle, combine ongoing daily estrogen for 3 months with 12 days of progesterone once every 3 months. Although they can lead to heavier and more painful withdrawal bleeding, they can be useful for women who are sensitive to the side effects of progesterone. When a woman is postmenopausal (no period for a year), continuous combined HRT can be prescribed.[23] Both hormones are taken daily so that there is no withdrawal bleeding.

Additional hormonal treatments include bazedoxifene and testosterone. Bazedoxifene is a combination medication containing estrogen and a selective estrogen receptor modulator. It is available in the United Kingdom and the United States and can be used in women who cannot tolerate progestogen; however, there are few long-term safety data.[28] Testosterone can also be used in addition to systemic HRT for women with androgen-related menopausal symptoms. These include low libido, low mood, and lack of energy.[4] At this time there are no licensed preparations for women, so it is an off-label therapy in the United States and an off-license preparation in the United Kingdom. It is generally given in addition to nonoral estrogen.[4,6,23]

In general, women without a uterus are able to take estrogen-only HRT. This lowers the risks of breast cancer.[4] The exception is women who have a hysterectomy due to severe endometriosis, because estrogen only can activate any deposits left in the pelvis.[6] In women with a partial hysterectomy, where a cervical stump was left behind, a trial of a sequential HRT to see if withdrawal bleeding occurs is needed.[6]

HORMONE REPLACEMENT THERAPY RISKS AND BENEFITS
Cardiovascular Disease

If HRT is started within the window of opportunity around the time of menopause or within 10 years of the LMP, the risk for CVD or cerebrovascular disease is considered low. Recent research and guidelines[4,6,23,25] contradict the Women's Health Initiative study of the early 2000s and now demonstrate that HRT is protective if used within this limited timeframe. HRT is cardioprotective in vitro and NICE states that HRT is the best treatment of VMSs and low mood related to menopause.[4]

Clotting Risks

Transdermal HRT has low or no risks of VTE compared with oral HRT,[4] whereas oral HRT in either a combined form or as estrogen only raises the risk. There is no impact from vaginal estrogens.[4]

Furthermore, there seems to be no increase in stroke if HRT is started early in menopause and less if transdermal therapy is used.[4]

Breast Cancer

HRT use has been associated with an increased risk of breast cancer and the risk increases with prolonged use.[4] This does not seem to be the case, however, with the use of estrogen only.[4] This observation led to studies looking at the different progesterone components within HRT to try to discover an optimum progesterone, with a lower risk profile. Women should be advised that there is an increased risk of breast cancer over and above their own background risk. This risk is actually lower than those with obesity and drinking alcohol.[29]

Stopping Hormone Replacement Therapy

There are no specific guidelines as to when a woman needs to stop HRT. Women should be counseled on the risks and benefits once a year if on an established HRT regimen (**Box 5**). Once a decision to stop is made, there is no clear advantage to stopping abruptly versus a gradual decrease.[4] It seems reasonable, however, to reduce to the lowest dose and then reassess for symptoms before stopping. If longer-term use is needed for older women, a transdermal preparation with female-friendly progestogens is the safest when considering cardiovascular and VTE risks.[6]

Side Effects

The main drawback of HRT can be the side effects and these can be divided into different categories (**Table 2**). When starting HRT, it is important to ensure that the woman has reasonable and realistic expectations about how HRT works, which symptoms it may help, and the time frame for relief. It is also important to discuss that sometimes she may need to try a few HRT combinations before she finds one that suits her. She should be followed-up at 3 months and then yearly once established on an acceptable treatment regimen.[4]

PREMATURE OVARIAN INSUFFICIENCY

Women can have menopause at any age. The definition of POI is menopause in any woman under the age of 40 (estimated to be approximately 1%),[30–32] whereas premature menopause is defined as cessation of menses in women under the age of 45. These definitions vary slightly in different countries. There are many guidelines for the management of this special group of women.[4,5,30] Despite these guidelines, women struggle to gain access to specialist services and to get a correct diagnosis because they are considered too young for menopause. Women who have amenorrhea need to be investigated by assessing the levels of FSH/LH/estradiol/prolactin. Additional tests are dependent on the results of initial levels of ovarian and pituitary hormones. Some women may have elevated FSH levels but continue to have normal menstrual cycles during the perimenopausal phase, which can last for a few years. To

---

Box 5
Benefits of hormone replacement therapy

- Effective treatment of VMSs and psychological symptoms
- Positive effects on urogenital symptoms and sexual function
- Effective treatment of mood
- Possible CVD protection
- Prevention of osteoporosis
- Possible effect on cognition
- Reduction in colorectal cancer

Table 2
Hormone replacement therapy side effects and problem solving

Estrogen Related	Progesterone Related	Method Related	Bleeding
HRT side effects			
• Breast tenderness • Nausea • Fluid retention • Headaches	• Moods/depression • Headaches • Skin issues • Libido • Fluid retention	• Skin irritation (patches) • Nausea (tablets)	• Monitor for first 6 mo
Problem solving			
• Lowest dose • Change delivery method • Change type of estrogen	• Change type of progesterone • Change delivery method • Use micronized progesterone or and IUS • Use tissue selective estrogen complex	• Change from patch to transdermal gel • Change from tablets to transdermal	• If investigations normal, change delivery method or dose • Consider IUS

establish a diagnosis of POI, women need to have at least 2 hormone profiles taken 4 weeks to 6 weeks apart. In addition, prolactin, thyroid-stimulating hormone, autoantibodies for thyroid adrenal studies, genetic evaluation for karyotyping and fragile X syndrome, and bone density (dual energy x-ray absorptiometry [DEXA]) are important to rule out other treatable causes and to establish baseline data.[3]

The causes of POI are varied. In most women, the cause it is unknown, but ongoing research is exploring the possibility of genetic causes.[7] There are factors that can cause an earlier menopause, such as smoking.[6] The most common causes are shown in **Box 6**.

Whatever the cause of POI, women need specialist care to help them manage symptoms.[4,5,30] Women often struggle with the diagnosis and lack peer support; thus, they may benefit from counseling for coping with the diagnosis and with the loss of fertility. A referral to a fertility specialist can be helpful to outline the possibilities of spontaneous pregnancy (5%–10%)[30] as can options for ovum donation, surrogacy, and adoption. In the United Kingdom, there is limited funding for infertility services for women with POI, and in the United States even with health insurance, care is costly. Women who have POI as a result of cancer, or who are about to begin chemotherapy,

Box 6
Causes of premature ovarian insufficiency

- Autoimmune disease
- Genetic (fragile X syndrome)
- Infection (mumps, tuberculosis)
- Chemotherapy
- Radiotherapy
- Surgical removal of ovaries

should be given the opportunity to discuss fertility options, such as egg/sperm freezing or freezing fertilized ovum.[3,5] Managing the long-term consequences of POI, such as osteoporosis, CVD, and higher mortality, is essential.[4,5,30]

Women with POI often have difficulty accessing accurate information about the use of HRT in their age group. Health care providers do not have access to studies involving women who are in this age group, which results in an unknown long-term risk prediction. Currently it is believed that there is no increased risk of cancer related to HRT until taken past the age of natural menopause.[30]

Once diagnosed, treatment should be offered for symptoms and for long-term health benefits, such as CVD and bone protection. It is important to discuss that HRT is not a contraceptive.[30] HRT may have a more protective role in bone preservation and against CVD than the option of the combined oral contraceptive pills.[3] This choice normally depends, however, on a woman's preference.

Regardless of treatment status, bone health should be assessed by DEXA scans at regular intervals. Women need advice on bone loss, diet, calcium, vitamin D, smoking, alcohol, and exercise. Women with POI may need an increased dosage of HRT, such as 4 mg orally or 100 mg transdermal, for symptom control and to assure ongoing adequate bone density. Women with POI should be kept under review until at least age 51 to 52.[30]

SPECIAL CONSIDERATION

Women who need special consideration are women with comorbidities. These include women who have an induced menopause, whether related to cancer or benign gynecological reasons, as well as women with POI. Often women who present for care with menopause symptoms have other conditions or comorbidities that need to be considered. **Table 3** lists some common concerns.

Women who have had cancer of the uterus, ovaries, cervix, or breast often experience menopause prematurely. In these women, there is an obvious concern about taking hormones. There are limited evidence and guidelines for their management, and a multidisciplinary approach is required, which, at minimum, should include a menopause specialist and an oncologist. There is some consensus for HRT use after certain cancers (**Table 4**).

NURSES AND THEIR ROLE IN MENOPAUSE

Nurses are in a prime position to see and advise women during menopause. Within the NICE guidance, women with certain conditions, such as cancer or previous VTE, should be referred for specialist services.[4] There is no definition on who qualifies as a specialist.[33] In the United Kingdom, there is no distinction between a medical or nurse specialist, and the Royal College of Nursing has developed guidance for nurses who wish to specialize in the care of menopausal women. This encompasses the 4 pillars of advanced practice[34]: clinical practice, leadership and management, education, and research.[35] In addition, at whatever level nurses are working, they should be able to direct women to appropriate sources of evidence and help. For example, in the United Kingdom, women should be directed to the Daisy Network (for POI, https://www.daisynetwork.org.uk/); Royal College of Obstetricians and Gynaecologists menopause hub (https://www.rcog.org.uk/en/patients/menopause/); Menopause Matters (https://menopausematters.co.uk/); Manage My Menopause (https://www.managemymenopause.co.uk/), British Menopause Society (https://thebms.org.uk), and Women's Health Concern (https://www.womens-health-concern.org/).

Table 3
Hormone replacement therapy and medical conditions

Condition	Advice
Fibroids	HRT is indicated but fibroids do not shrink. If bleeding is a problem, suggest IUS and estrogen.
Endometriosis	Sequential HRT may reactivate deposits (IUS and estrogen best); if posthysterectomy, continuous combined HRT prevents reactivation of residual disease.
Hypertension	Transdermal preferred
Migraines	Combined continuous HRT preferred; if perimenopausal, try IUS and patch or gel of estrogen.
Bowel issues	Avoid oral
Benign breast disease	Common side effect
Diabetes	Monitor/manage risk factors; if under control, HRT may be used; transdermal has less impact on control of blood sugars and is safer if other risk factors exist.
Epilepsy	Nonoral
HIV	Consider interactions of multiple medications; evidence suggests earlier menopause.
BRCA	Data limited but tend to suggest HRT is ok until natural age of menopause if post–risk reduction surgery.
VTE	Investigate, refer to specialist; transdermal may be safe.
Thyroid	Thyroxine may need to be increased if on oral HRT.

DIFFERENCES BETWEEN THE UNITED KINGDOM AND THE UNITED STATES

The menopause symptoms that women experience are the same for many women in the United Kingdom and the United States; in addition, the lifestyle changes that women need to make are similar. Both countries have menopause societies, but in the United Kingdom, the management of menopause, both in primary community care and specialist secondary care, is covered under the NHS. In both countries, women pay for most prescriptions. The age of menopause is not significantly different between the United Kingdom and the United States (age 51–52). The range, however, is variable, with the United Kingdom at 45 to 56 years old and the United States at 40 to 58 years old.[36]

The principles of care and management are similar but some medications differ. The United Kingdom prescribes less conjugated equine estrogen. The guidelines and risks

Table 4
Cancer and hormone replacement therapy

Cancer	Research/Guidance
Ovarian	Acceptable but limited data on endometroid[7]
Cervical	Squamous cell cancer has no link with HRT; use with caution for a history of adenocarcinoma.
Vulva	HRT not contraindicated
Endometrial	Depends on the type and stage
Breast	Depends on hormonal status of the cancer; in general, HRT not recommended in hormone sensitive lesion (unless other treatments have failed and quality of life severely impacted).

and benefits are broadly in line in both countries.[37] Both countries also have the opportunity for nurses to enhance and expand their role in menopause care.

SUMMARY

Nurses are in a good position to talk to and educate women about menopause and related issues. All nurses see women in menopause regardless of their field of specialty and in addition see colleagues who have menopausal symptoms. Menopause is a minefield of different symptoms and varying treatments, and it is difficult to keep on top of the latest guidance but essential to have a balanced and evidenced-based view to enable women to live in a healthy postmenopausal state.

REFERENCES

1. Rossouw JE, Anderson GL, Prentice RL, et al. Risks and benefits of estrogen plus progestin in healthy postmenopausal women: principal results from the Women's Health Initiative randomized controlled trial. J Am Med Assoc 2002;288(3): 321–33.
2. Million Women Study Collaborators. Breast cancer and hormone-replacement therapy in the Million Women Study. Lancet 2003;326(9382):419–27.
3. Maki P, Duffecy J. An e- Health approach to treating vasomotor symptoms. Menopause 2017;24(7):722–3.
4. Available at: https://www.nice.org.uk/guidance/NG23. Accessed September 22, 2017.
5. Available at: https://www.nice.org.uk/guidance/qs143. Accessed September 22, 2017.
6. Hillard T, Abernethy K, Hamoda H, et al, editors. Management of the menopause. The handbook. 6th edition. London (United Kingdom): British Menoapsual Society; 2017.
7. Laven J, Visser J, Uittlind A, et al. Menopause: genome stability as new paradigm. Maturitas 2016;92:15–23.
8. Baber R. The hot flush: symptom or sign of disease. Climacteric 2017;20(4): 291–2.
9. National Institute for Health and Care Excellence Guideline Suspected cancer: recognition and referral [NICE, 2015]. Available at: https://www.nice.org.uk/guidance/ng12.
10. Timmermans A, Opmeer BC, Khan KS, et al. Endometrial thickness measurement for detecting endometrial cancer in women with postmenopausal bleeding: a systematic review and meta-analysis. Obstet Gynecol 2010;116(1):160–7. Available at: http://www.crd.york.ac.uk/crdweb/PrintPDF.php?AccessionNumber=12010008039& Copyright=Database+of+Abstracts+of+Reviews+of+Effects+%28DARE%29% 3Cbr+%2F%3EProduced+by+the+Centre+for+Reviews+and+Dissemination+ %3Cbr+%2F%3ECopyright+%26copy%3B+2017+University+of+York%3Cbr+ %2F%3E.
11. 2011. Available at: https://www.rcog.org.uk/globalassets/documents/guidelines/ gtg59hysteroscopy.pdf. Accessed September 22, 2017.
12. Wysocki S, Kingsberg S, Krychman M. Management of vaginal atrophy: implications from the REVIVE survey. Clin Med Insights Reprod Health 2014;8:23–30.
13. Gartoulla P, Bell R, Worsley R, et al. Menopausal vasomotor symptoms are associated with poor self-assessed work ability. Maturitas 2016;87:33–9.

14. Hardy C, Griffiths A, Hunter M. What do working menopausal women want? A qualitative investigation into women's perspectives on employer and line manager support. Maturitas 2017;101:37–41.
15. Available at: https://www.fsrh.org/standards-and-guidance/documents/fsrh-guidance-contraception-for-women-aged-over-40-years-2017/. Accessed September 22, 2017.
16. Nonhormonal management of menopause-associated vasomotor symptoms: 2015 position statement of the North American menopause society. Menopause 2015;22(11):1155–72.
17. Woyka J. Consensus statement for non-hormonal based treatments for menopausal symptoms. Post Reprod Health 2017;23(2):71–5.
18. Mintziori G, Lamrinoudaki I, Goulis D, et al. EMAS position statement: non-hormonal management of menopausal vasomotor symptoms. Maturitas 2015; 81(3):410–3.
19. Cochran CJ, Gallicchio L, Miller SR, et al. Cigarette smoking, androgen levels, and hot flushes in midlife women. Obstet Gynecol 2008;112(5):1037–44.
20. Sassarini J, Anderson R. New pathways in the treatment for menopause hot flushes. Lancet 2017;389:1775–7.
21. Desmarais JE, Looper KJ. Managing menopausal symptoms and depression in tamoxifen users: implications of drug and medicinal interactions. Maturitas 2010;67:296–308.
22. Kaunitz A, Pinkerton J, Manson J. Menopause. OBG Management 2017;29(6): 18–24.
23. Hamoda H, Panay N, Arya R, et al, on behalf the British Menopause Society and Women's Health Concern. Recommendations on HRT in menopausal women. Post Reprod Health 2016;22(4):165–83.
24. Arroyo C. Fractional CO_2 laser treatment for vulvovaginal atrophy symptoms and vaginal rejuvenation in perimenopausal women. Int J Womens Health 2017;9: 591–5.
25. Available at: https://thebms.org.uk/2017/03/bms-council-issues-consensus-statement-bioidentical-hormones/. Accessed September 22, 2017.
26. L'Hermite M. Custom compound bio-identical hormone therapy-why so popular despite potential harm? The case against routine use. Climacteric 2017;20(3): 205–11.
27. Mikkola T, Savolainen-pekoski H, Venetkoski M, et al. New evidence for cardiac benefit of post-menopausal hormone therapy. Climacteric 2017;20(1):5–10.
28. Bazedoxifene for HRT. Drug Ther Bull 2017;55:42–4.
29. Available at: https://thebms.org.uk/_wprs/wp-content/uploads/2016/04/WHC-UnderstandingRisksofBreastCancer-MARCH2017.pdf. Accessed September 22, 2017.
30. Hamoda H, on behalf of the British Menopause Society and Women's Health Concern. The British Menopause Society and Women's Health Concern recommendations on the management of women with premature ovarian insufficiency. Post Reprod Health 2017;23(1):22–35.
31. Guideline of the European Society of Human reproduction and embryology. Management of women with premature ovarian insufficiency. 2015. Available at: https://www.eshre.eu/Guidelines-and-Legal/Guidelines/Management-of-premature-ovarian-insufficiency.aspx.
32. Available at: https://www.rcn.org.uk/professional-development/publications/pub-005986. Accessed September 22, 2017.

33. Available at: https://thebms.org.uk/menopause-specialists/overview/. Accessed September 22, 2017.
34. Available at: https://www.rcn.org.uk/professional-development/publications/pub-005701. Accessed September 22, 2017.
35. Manley K. A conceptual framework for advanced practice: an action research project operationalising an advanced practitioner/nurse consultant role. J Clin Nurs 1997;6(3):179–90.
36. Available at: http://www.menopause.org/publications/clinical-care-recommendations/chapter-1-menopause. Accessed September 22, 2017.
37. Available at: http://www.menopause.org/docs/default-source/2017/nams-2017-hormone-therapy-position-statement.pdf. Accessed September 22, 2017.

Sexuality and Intimacy in the Older Adult Woman

Alice L. March, RN, PhD, FNP, CNE

KEYWORDS

- Older women • Sexuality • Sexual behaviors • Intimacy

KEY POINTS

- Although one in every 5 older adults reports recent sexual activity, health care professionals do not typically ask older people about sexual intimacy.
- Only one in 5 women discussed sexual concerns with their professional after the age of 50.
- Practitioners may lack education and comfort related to communication about sexuality.
- An effective means of communication and assessment is the PLISSIT model.

Adults over 65 years old are more likely to seek health care than persons less than 65 years old. In the United States, this equates to approximately 248 million visits each year or 7 visits per older adult annually.[1] Although one in every 5 older adults reports recent sexual activity,[2] health care professionals do not typically ask about sexual intimacy, and patients are often reluctant to bring the matter to the attention of the examiner for a variety of reasons.[3,4] Several factors may contribute to a lack of discussion of sexuality when caring for older adult women. Some of these include (1) societal perceptions that older women are not having sex, (2) health care professionals fear insulting the woman by asking personal questions, or (3) practitioners may be uncomfortable discussing sexual intimacy with women who may be the same age as their own parents or grandparents.[3] Regardless of the rationale for this lack of assessment, the end result is that older adults may have unmet needs related to sexual intimacy.[4,5]

FACTS, MYTHS, AND SOCIOCULTURAL INFLUENCES

There are potential problems surrounding assessing the extent of intimate behaviors in older women. The frequency of sexual activity declines as adults age, yet many older women desire and have the capacity for sexual activity.[2,3,6,7] The desire for sex and physical intimacy is influenced by several aspects, including relationship status, caregiving responsibilities, and the health status of the partner.[8] Even with all these variables at work, women in the United States report the following percentages of

Dr A.L. March has no financial interests to disclose.
Capstone College of Nursing, The University of Alabama, Box 870358, 650 University Boulevard, Tuscaloosa, AL 35401, USA
E-mail address: almarch@ua.edu

sexual activity: 51% during their 60s, 30% in their 70s, and 20% in their 80s.[9] Intimacy behaviors that do not require significant physical functionality and/or stamina may occur at a higher percent, yet these numbers are unknown. It is also difficult to know the prevalence of sexual problems. In one study, half of the sexually active older men and women reported at least one sexual concern or problem, and women were more likely to report at least 2 problems.[10]

As women age, the percent of women who are sexually active decreases; however, age is only one factor affecting behavior. Among these are functional status and culture. As functional status declines, the number of sexual problems increases.[10] Cultural influences and minority identities contribute to attitudes, experiences, and perceived needs related to sexual intimacy and may also alter attitudes about sharing sexual information with health care professionals.[11] The composition of older adult demographics is rapidly becoming more diverse, and the influences of religion, politics, and historical events shape worldviews and result in formation of the values and mores related to sexual intimacy.[11] A prime example of historical influence is the effect of the sexual revolution on an older generation referred to as Baby Boomers who significantly changed views on casual sexual relations.[10,12,13] Women who are older than Baby Boomers (born before 1945) may be more conservative in their views and practices related to sexuality and may be less likely to initiate communication with health care professionals.[14]

Satisfaction with one's sexual life is affected by many factors, some known[15] and some unknown. Facts and myths about aging and sexuality are influenced by societal views concerning who should and who should not be participating in intimate behaviors. These beliefs continue to influence attitudes related to intimacy in older women, despite the positive outcomes provided by sexual satisfaction.[6,15,16] The positive effects of satisfaction with the status of one's sexual life, whether or not able to achieve sexual intercourse, are listed in **Box 1**.[15]

Intimacy is influenced by several internal and external factors. These factors include (1) cognition, (2) biology, and (3) psychosocial elements.[6] Spiritual beliefs play a significant role in how older women view sexuality.[2] Historically, because of religious influences, some cultures held an underlying belief that sex was solely for procreation,[9] and enjoyment was not valued, and perhaps even self-indulgent. As such, it was believed that older women should not continue such activities. This belief is countered by a more recent social change, the trend to use medication and therapies to allow sexual behaviors despite age or disability.[6]

A major part of sexual identity is how women experience the human body and her perceptions regarding the body.[17] Sexual identity has a bearing on intimacy, and past behaviors are predictive of what occurs at older ages.[4,17] Although the frequency of sex declines with age, a sizable number of older adults continue intimate activities up to age 90.[4] What is not known is the frequency and types of behaviors after age 90. Intimate relationships may be more satisfying when linked with the closeness associated with hugging, kissing, caressing, and hand holding before intercourse.[4] Older adults who expressed contentment with their sexual life reported many factors that contribute to this satisfaction. Several factors are included in **Box 2**.[18]

Box 1
The effects of sexual satisfaction

1. Predicts positive perception of health and well-being

2. Contributes to quality of life

3. Importance spiritual and religious influence

Box 2
Factors related to sexual satisfaction

1. A sexual partner
2. Frequent sexual intercourse
3. Good health
4. Low levels of stress
5. Absence of financial worries

Viewing one's self as an attractive sexual being and functional intimate partner is influenced by societal norms. Advertising clearly emphasizes that intimate behaviors and sexual activity are for young, attractive people, as demonstrated by using young healthy people for product endorsements.[4,9] Advertisers typically do not focus on older individuals, unless the product is directly related to that specific population. In addition, there is an aging double standard. Product placement is more likely to present desirable women as young, in contrast to sexually attractive men who may be portrayed as middle aged, or even older.[9] As a result, the societal impact from advertising shapes beliefs, attitudes, emotions, and actions related to sexual intimacy and behaviors.[17] Regardless of how most older adults are portrayed in the media and viewed by society, a continued desire for intimacy exists.

DEBUNKING THE MYTHS

The desire to engage in sex and intimate behaviors to meet important quality-of-life needs is present in people of all ages.[3,16] Intimacy is defined as an emotional response to being loved and cared for.[9] This intimacy includes both physical and emotional intimacy and considers the influence of sexual experience, attitudes, character, expression, and actions.[4] Sexual intimacy, included within the broader realm of intimacy, may focus on emotional closeness as well as the physical act of intercourse. Intimacy and intimate encounters include not just sexual intercourse but also cuddling, petting, and genital stimulation, as well as the emotional or physical touch of another human.[19]

An important aspect of sexual intimacy is the presence of a partner available to engage in these behaviors.[6] It is common for women who experienced long-term monogamous relationships to lose an intimate partner, yet still desire sexual intimacy. In the United States, the percent of older adults living in a married relationship (with a spouse present) varies by gender with a growing disparity between men and women as age increases.[6] For women age 65 years or older, 41% are married, 44% are widowed, and 9% are divorced.[20] For men aged 65 years or more, 71% are married, 14% are widowed, and 7% are divorced. These figures do not reflect living arrangements of adults living together apart, nor do they include gay, lesbian, or other nontraditional couples (lesbian, gay, bisexual, transgender, or questioning [LGBTQ]).

THE REAL ISSUE: BIOPHYSICAL ASPECTS AND THE IMPACT OF ILLNESS

When considering the challenges faced by older women related to sexual intimacy, the biophysical aspect of aging must be examined. Normal age-related anatomic changes and decreasing hormone levels occur, and because of these changes, a slower sexual response is experienced. Sexual changes in women from declining female hormones result in greater bladder and urethral irritation, increased risk of infection, less vaginal lubrication, changes in orgasms, and loss of pleasure during intercourse.[6,16,21,22]

The lack of estrogen results in thinning of the vaginal wall, and a decrease in the onset and amount of lubrication. Without intervention (ie, use of lubricant), this results in inflamed and irritated tissues leading to uncomfortable or painful intercourse. In addition, there is a decrease in the ability to reach orgasm, and the intensity is often lessened, thus, decreasing the overall desire to have sexual intercourse.[6,9,16]

The physiologic process of aging (vaginal dryness and thinning of tissue) increases the risk of transmission of sexually transmitted infections (STIs), including HIV/AIDS. The aging immune system may not be as able to prevent transmission.[23] Older women report a lack of concern about pregnancy, and therefore, they are not as likely to consider condom use to be a priority issue. Menopausal women may not be taking estrogen; thus, the thinner, less healthy, and less well-lubricated vaginal tissue has an increased potential for tissue disruption and risk for transmission of many STIs. In addition, the cervix undergoes changes that are particularly favorable to the transmission of HIV.[24]

To make matters worse, older women often have no symptoms of STIs, or they present to health care providers with menopausal symptoms, such as pelvic pain, deep dyspareunia, and postcoital bleeding, which may actually be chlamydia and gonorrhea. About one in 3 cases of STIs is detected by yearly screening procedures, rather than the presentation of symptoms. The loss of estrogen with the subsequent friability and atrophy of tissue may also result in a missed diagnosis of herpes by presenting as vulvar ulcerations, soreness, or dysuria.[25] An additional STI concern is related to risk for cervical and vulvar cancers due to human papillomavirus infection. Women are not using barrier methods, have age-related immune changes, and do not routinely seek Pap smears. In many cases, insurance companies do not cover the cost or are reluctant to pay for these on a regular basis.[26] This combination of factors places older women at risk for advanced disease at time of diagnosis.

Multiple physical changes or chronic health conditions occur in 69% of persons age 65 years or older. These health issues lead to disability and impact sexual intimacy.[3,12] The presence of hypertension, high cholesterol, arthritis, back problems, diabetes, and depression decreases quality of life and affects the desire for intimacy and for intercourse.[27] In addition, these health alterations decrease enjoyment of everyday life, worsen mobility (making positioning a challenge), or lessen activity tolerance.[28] For women, changes in body image as normal aging occurs, or after a mastectomy or other surgical procedure (ie, open heart), may decrease comfort with disrobing. Medical conditions accelerate changes in aging bodies, and this also adversely affects the desire for physical intimacy.[28]

HEALTH CARE PROFESSIONALS' ASSESSMENT AND COMMUNICATION

The literature on communication between patients and health care professionals is scant; however, in one study only one in 5 (22%) women discussed sexual concerns with their professional after the age of 50.[2] Multiple reasons for this exist. Health care professionals do not ask, and older persons do not tell. The sexual histories and practices of older women are not routinely collected for a variety of reasons. Elders are perceived to be at low risk for STIs, including HIV/AIDS, and health care professionals may be emotionally uncomfortable discussing sexual issues with women for reasons listed above.[5] Because the presentation of STIs and HIV in women with multiple chronic diseases may significantly change the expected presentation, practitioners are confounded. In addition, the time allotted for a visit is spent reviewing current status and medications, and new changes may be ascribed to other causes (medication effects and disease progression) by both the professional and the patient.[29]

Because it is important to communicate in a nonjudgmental manner, health care professionals must first examine their own personal attitudes and values regarding sexuality in older women. This type of introspection will lead to more comfort in conversations about intimate behaviors and may facilitate discussions about other underlying concerns.[3,17] It is essential to have a thorough understanding of the expected physical aging changes, the potential effects of chronic medical conditions, and medications on sexual function. It is also important to understand that aging does not occur at the same rate in all women, and women may not perceive themselves "old."[3]

Assessing the importance of intimacy and intercourse for each woman is a starting point for the health care professional, who may be uncertain about discussing these issues. Subtle cues must be recognized and acted on to begin communication about potential problems.[17,22] Once cues are identified, clear nonmedical terms must be used to describe sexual behaviors. It may be beneficial to open the discussion in terms of less personal questions, or to inquire about a sequence of events or stories related to the older woman's personal sexual history.[3,17] For example, it may seem less personally threatening to the older woman if the health care professional asks about foreplay, kissing, holding hands, or verbal expression of affection as intimate behaviors.[17]

Communication is critical when addressing sexual intimacy needs. Multiple areas of inquiry exist. Inquiring about the physical comfort of intercourse and other sexual behaviors is important, but asking about the psychological and emotional level of comfort is equally important. Educating the woman about how medical conditions and medications used to treat those diseases affect sexual responses (important for lubrication and thus comfort) is another topic for discussion.[30]

An effective means of communication and assessment is the PLISSIT model, which uses open-ended questions to explore concerns. PLISSIT is an acronym for the levels of the model's intervention (**Table 1**).[31]

The P, which is the first step in the model, represents permission. Permission has 2 components. First, it requires the health care professional to ask permission to discuss sex and intimate behaviors. Second, the health care professional gives the older woman reassurance (permission to believe) that her thoughts, fears, and desires are normal.[28] This permission creates a feeling of control for the patient and for the partner (if present).

The second step in the model is LI (limited information). The interaction should contain limited information that is directly related to the expressed problem. When applicable, it may be necessary to discuss the normal anatomy and physiology of sexual functioning as it relates to the aging process, current medications (of both partners), and chronic conditions.[28] It is important to use nonmedical terms, but at the same time not use inappropriate or demeaning terms. Listening to the terms used by the woman helps guide the practitioner during discussion and when offering the information.

The third step in the approach is SS (specific suggestions).[28] Suggestions relate directly back to the answers to the open-ended questions, and options for those

Table 1	
Content of the PLISST model	
P	Permission
LI	Limited information
SS	Specific suggestions
IT	Intensive therapy

Box 3
Recommendations to improve sexual intimacy
1. Think about when and where to have sex
2. Be rested and relaxed
3. Take pain medication about 2 hours before
4. Consider alternate sexual activities
5. Remember intimacy takes other forms, including touching and hugging
6. Be an effective communicator
7. Use special aids and equipment if needed
8. Place a personal emphasis on comfort, warmth, and joy
9. Be positive and affirming
From Fisher L. Sex, romance, and relationships. AARP survey of midlife and older adults. Washington, DC: American Association of Retired People; 2010. Publication D19234; with permission.

suggestions should be presented. Health literacy must be considered and specific suggestions should be simple and direct. Suggestions might include pictures of positions and written exercises in large font. When possible, take time to discuss the written material and use the teach-back method to ensure understanding. If time is limited during that visit, consider a follow-up visit to check progress.

Intensive therapy (IT) is the final component, and in most cases, the woman will not need this approach. However, the health care professional should be prepared to make appropriate referrals when long-term therapy is warranted, for example, in cases directly related to functional decline that might respond to physical or occupation therapy, true sexual dysfunction not due to normal aging, or relationship issues.[28]

INTERVENTION CONSIDERATIONS

Aging takes place across a continuum of settings, including the private homes of older women (or their children), assisted living, and skilled nursing facilities. Couples may not reside in the same physical building or at the same level of care, and it is reasonable to consider how the opportunity for sexual intimacy could be provided. Recommendations to improve sexual intimacy can be given to all older adults (**Box 3**), but for many, privacy is the most significant factor.[11]

Box 4
Barriers to sexual intimacy in institutionalized older women
1. Personal beliefs, education, and values of staff
2. Family dynamics
3. Education level of woman (and family)
4. Partner availability and ability
5. Physical disabilities
6. Sexual orientation
7. Diminished cognition (woman or partner)

Table 2
Interprofessional approaches to sexual dysfunction

Physical therapy	Increase mobility and stamina
Occupational therapy	Assistance with positioning, energy conservation, and adaptive aids
Rehabilitation specialist/sexual therapist	Optimize functioning by minimizing disabilities or impairments and maximizing societal participation

The residential location of an older woman has major implications on how sexuality is perceived, accepted, and expressed. Location may be a special challenge for those living in communal settings or with family members.[7] In older adults who are LGBTQ, these challenges are compounded by societal constraints placed on the open expression of intimacy; however, little research exists because older adults who are LGBTQ may be hesitant to identify themselves.[10] In addition to a strong potential for lack of privacy, barriers related to sexual intimacy in institutionalized older adults are listed in **Box 4**.[4,12]

Displays of sexual intimacy by older women, whether in the community or living in long-term care settings, may be regarded as inappropriate behavior by staff or family, especially when the older woman has any level of cognitive impairment.[19] Institutions may have policies that deny or restrict the sexuality intimacy of residents, and in addition to those restrictions, residents are likely to lack privacy.[17] Because it may be difficult for families and older women to broach this sensitive subject, one solution is a proactive approach to initiate the discussion.[32] This proactive approach can be accomplished using the PLISST model.

Health care professionals must work as a team to recognize sexual intimacy concerns, and to deal with them within the scope of their profession or make appropriate referrals.[32] Rather than setting limits on intercourse or intimacy expression, the focus should be on developing a balance of autonomy and safety to facilitate intimacy, perhaps by providing permission and privacy.[17] Educating staff and families about the sexual needs of older women and encouraging support and arrangements for sexual intimacy is one place to begin.

Sexual dysfunction is more common in the presence of chronic disease, cancer, or other physical impairments, thus, requiring holistic and differing approaches. Older women may not be able to benefit from the simple and general recommendations that address sexual intimacy, but instead may need a multidimensional care approach. Interventions should be considered from an interprofessional lens, as noted in **Table 2**.[21,32,33]

SUMMARY

Health care professionals are integral to assessing and managing normal and pathologic aging changes impacting the quality of life for older women.[27] Sexual dysfunction is one issue that may reduce quality of life, may cause marital problems, may diminish self-esteem, and may be clinically manifested in the form of depression, anxiety, tension, and hypochondria complaints.[21] It is important to assess barriers to sexual intercourse and intimacy whether they are physiologic, psychosocial, or environmental in nature. To meet the sexual needs of older women, it is vitally important that issues related to sexual intimacy are openly discussed during health care encounters. Health care professionals who feel they do not have adequate education in these matters should seek continuing education opportunities. In addition, for those who are uncomfortable with sexual questions, they should practice in the mirror or with colleagues. Creating and carrying a pocket card of the PLISST model can be a helpful memory aid.

To provide holistic care, health care professionals must develop an appreciation for diversity and how this impacts the expression of sexual intimacy in older women. Prudent assessment practices include a comprehensive sexual health history and assessment to determine the presence or absence of sexual intimacy concerns.[11] Older women are not asexual beings; yet culturally induced embarrassment, fear, and anxiety are important factors in the decision to disclose problem or behaviors.[34]

REFERENCES

1. American Association of Colleges of Nursing. Recommended baccalaureate competencies and curricular guidelines for the nursing care of older adults. Available at: http://www.aacnnursing.org/Portals/42/AcademicNursing/CurriculumGuidelines/AACN-Gero-Competencies-2010.pdf?ver=2017-05-18-132343-233. Accessed November 1, 2017.
2. Lindau ST, Schumm LP, Laumann EO, et al. A study of sexuality and health among older adults in the United States. N Engl J Med 2007;357:762–74.
3. Sarkisian CA, Hays RD, Berry SH, et al. Expectations regarding aging among older adults and physicians who care for older adults. Med Care 2001;39: 1025–36.
4. Hillman J. A call for integrated biopsychosocial model to address fundamental disconnects in an emergent field: an introduction to the special issue on "sexuality and aging". Ageing Int 2011;36:303–12.
5. Loeb DF, Lee RS, Binswanger IA, et al. Patient, resident physician, and visit factors associated with documentation of sexual history in the outpatient setting. J Gen Intern Med 2011;26:887–93.
6. DeLamater JD, Sill M. Sexual desire in later life. J Sex Res 2005;42:138–49.
7. Jagus CE, Benbow SM. Sexuality in older men with mental health problems. Sex Relation Ther 2002;17:271–9.
8. Fileborn B, Thorpe R, Hawkes G, et al. Sex, desire and pleasure: considering the experiences of Australian women. Sex Relation Ther 2015;30(1):117–30.
9. Crooks R, Baur K. Our sexuality. 11th edition. Belmont (CA): Wadsworth Cengage Learning; 2011.
10. Connolly MT, Breckman R, Callahan J, et al. The sexual revolution's last frontier: how silence about sex undermines health, well-being, and safety in old age. J Am Society on Aging 2012;36:43–52.
11. Orel NA, Watson WK. Addressing diversity in sexuality and aging: key considerations for healthcare providers. Available at: http://www.aginglifecarejournal.org/addressing-diversity-in-sexuality-and-aging-key-considerations-for-healthcare-providers/. Accessed November 1, 2018.
12. Yee L. Aging and sexuality. Aust Fam Physician 2010;39:718–21.
13. Fileborn B, Thorpe R, Hawkes G, et al. Sex and the older single girl: experiences of sex and dating in later life. J Aging Stud 2015;33:67–75.
14. Goodroad BK. HIV and AIDS in people older than 50: a continuing concern. J Gerontol Nurs 2003;29(4):18–24.
15. Weeks DJ. Sex for the mature adult: health, self-esteem, and countering ageist stereotypes. Sex Relation Ther 2002;17:231–40.
16. Bancroft J. Promoting sexual health and responsible sexual behavior. J Sex Res 2002;39:15–21.

17. Price B. Exploring attitudes towards older people's sexuality. Nurs Older People 2009;21:32–9.
18. Fisher L. Sex, romance, and relationships. AARP survey of midlife and older adults. Washington, DC: American Association of Retired People; 2010. Publication D19234.
19. Allen RS, Petro KN, Phillips LL. Factors influencing young adults' attitudes and knowledge of late-life sexuality among older women. Aging Ment Health 2009; 13:238–45.
20. He W, Sengupta M, Velkoff VV, et al. 65+ in the United States: 2005. Washington, DC: U.S. Government Printing Office; 2005.
21. Laftin M. Sexuality and elderly individual. In: Lewis CB, editor. Aging: the health-care challenge. Philadelphia: F.A. Davis; 2002. p. 278–300.
22. Hillman J. Sexual issues and aging within the context of work with older adult patients. Prof Psychol Res Pr 2008;39:290–7.
23. Nichols JE. Prevention of HIV disease in older adults. In: Emlet CA, editor. HIV/AIDS and older adults: challenges for individuals, families, and communities. New York: Springer; 2004. p. 21–36.
24. Rollenhagen C, Asin S. Enhanced HIV-1 replication in ex vivo ectocervical tissues from post-menopausal women correlates with increased inflammatory responses. Mucosal Immunol 2011;4(6):671–81.
25. Drew O, Sherrard J. Sexually transmitted infections in the older woman. Menopause Int 2008;14(3):134–5.
26. Minkin NJ. Sexually transmitted infections and the aging female: placing risks in perspective. Maturitas 2010;67:114–6.
27. American Association of Retired Persons (AARP). Sexuality at midlife and beyond. Washington, DC: American Association of Retired People; 2005.
28. Rheaume C, Mitty E. Sexuality and intimacy in older adults. Geriatr Nurs 2008;29: 342–9.
29. Siegel K, Lekas H-M, Schrimshaw EW, et al. Strategies adopted by late middle-age and older adults with HIV/AIDS to explain their physical symptoms. Psychol Health 2011;26(Supp1):41–62.
30. Slinkard MS, Wallace M. Older adults and HIV and STI screening: the patient perspective. Geriatr Nurs 2011;32(5):341–9.
31. Annon J. The PLISSIT model: a proposed conceptual scheme for the behavioral treatment of sexual problems. J Sex Educ Ther 1976;2:1–15.
32. Gianotten WL, Bender JL, Post MW, et al. Training in sexology for medical and paramedical professionals: a model for the rehabilitation setting. Sex Relation Ther 2006;21:303–17.
33. Tipton-Burton M. Occupational therapy: practice skills for physical dysfunction. St Louis (MO): Elsevier; 2013. p. 295–313.
34. Senelick R, Dougherty K. Living with stroke: a guide for families. 4th edition. Birmingham (AL): Healthsouth Press; 2010.

Person-Centered Care for Patients with Pessaries

Gwendolyn L. Hooper, PhD, FNP-BC, CUNP

KEYWORDS

- Pessary • Pelvic organ prolapse • Patient-centered care

KEY POINTS

- Pessaries are a safe and effective treatment option for women with pelvic organ prolapse.
- Family and cultural attitudes, beliefs, and perceptions can influence women's decisions for pessary use.
- Managing a patient with a pessary incorporates holistic and person-centered care.

INTRODUCTION

The pelvis of the human woman consists of a complex and intricate system of muscles, ligaments, nerves, and blood vessels. The pelvis houses the uterus and ovaries, stores the bladder and colon, and provides specific functions for sexual reproduction and childbirth. The muscles and ligaments of the pelvic floor support the internal organs of the pelvis by forming a structure similar to a trampoline. When the muscles and ligaments weaken, pelvic organ prolapse (POP) takes place, allowing the bladder, uterus, intestines, and/or support tissues to herniate into the vaginal opening.

To standardize terminology, physical findings, and enhance POP research, the International Urogynecological Association and International Continence Society define prolapse as "the descent of one or more of the anterior vaginal wall, posterior vaginal wall, the uterus (cervix) or the apex of the vagina (vaginal vault or cuff scar after hysterectomy)."[1] Several different types of prolapse occur in women, yet there is no universally accepted system for grading, staging, recording, or describing the support of the pelvic floor (Table 1).[2,3] To describe parameters of the pelvis for the appropriate fitting of a pessary, experts advocate for dividing the pelvis into anterior, posterior, middle, and apical compartments for clinical use.[4] Popular systems currently used for grading prolapse are the Baden-Walker and Pelvic Organ Prolapse Quantification System[5] (Table 2).

The author has nothing to disclose concerning commercial or financial conflicts of interest and received no funding regarding this article.
Graduate Nursing, Capstone College of Nursing, The University of Alabama, Box 870358, Tuscaloosa, AL 35487-0358, USA
E-mail address: glhooper@ua.edu

> **Box 1**
> **Treatment options**
>
> Pelvic floor muscle exercises
>
> Surgery
>
> Pessary
>
> No treatment if emptying bladder and bowel well and no bother to patient. Consider reevaluation at a later date if symptoms develop

EPIDEMIOLOGY OF PELVIC ORGAN PROLAPSE

Prolapse can occur in women of any age, racial, or ethnic group. Women ages 57 to 84 years old are more likely than other age group to present with this condition,[6,7] and the rates are similar regardless of the presence of the uterus (38%) versus no uterus (41%).[8] White women are at greater risk for POP than Black women.[9] The risk of POP with uterine prolapse is highest among Latino women, as opposed to Black women, who have the lowest risk.[8] Black women and white women are equally susceptible to the development of prolapse as a result of childbirth.[9–11]

Other risk factors for POP include body mass index, family history, chronic intra-abdominal pressure, genetic factors,[12] and childbirth history.[13] The number of full-term pregnancies, infant birth weight, and forceps delivery are important predictors.[13] Overweight and obese women are more likely than women with a normal body mass index to have POP.[14] Chronic repetitive straining (dyschezia), heavy lifting, and high-impact activity contribute to weakened muscles, ligaments, and connective tissue, leading to prolapse.[6] Teenagers who engage in strenuous activity have a greater occurrence of POP than middle-aged women who do not routinely engage in such behaviors.[6] Vaginal delivery is considered a risk factor[15–18]; however, elective cesarean section has been shown to be only partially effective in preventing POP.[11] Women with Ehlers-Danlos syndrome or Marfan syndrome have higher rates of pelvic floor disorders, including POP and urinary incontinence[19,20] (**Table 3**).

QUALITY OF LIFE IN WOMEN WITH PELVIC ORGAN PROLAPSE

Symptoms of prolapse are variable. Women report lower abdominal or pelvic pain, pressure, and heaviness[21]; limitations of body strength and mobility[11]; recurrent urinary tract infection; inability to place and retain a tampon; and dyspareunia. With severe prolapse, decubitus ulcer and excoriated tissues caused by the prolapse rubbing against skin, underwear, or protective pads can occur.[22]

Table 1	
Types of pelvic organ prolapse	
Cystocele	Descent of the bladder base below the ramus of the symphysis pubis, either at rest or with straining
Enterocele	Herniation of the peritoneum and its contents at the level of the vaginal apex.
Rectocele	An intravaginal herniation of the rectum through the rectovaginal septum
Uterine	Descent of the uterus at rest or straining

From Rosenblum N, Eilber KS, Rodriguez LV, et al. Anatomy of Pelvic Support. In: Appell RA, Sand PK, Raz S, editors. Female urology, urogynecology, and voiding dysfunction. Boca Raton (FL): Taylor and Francis; 2005; with permission.

Table 2	
Grades and descriptions of prolapse defined by Baden-Walker system	
G0	No prolapse
G1	Halfway to the hymen or remnant of the hymen
G2	To the introitus (the vaginal opening)
G3	Halfway past the hymen or remnant of the hymen
G4	Maximum descent

Abbreviation: G, grade of prolapse.
Data from Beckly I, Harris N. Pelvic organ prolapse: a urology perspective. J Clin Urol 2013;6(2):68–76.

POP can cause dramatic changes to the urogenital tract of women, creating a negative impact on perceived body image and physical and sexual attractiveness, thus leading to feelings of shame, embarrassment, and isolation.[23] Depression, also reported in women with POP dramatically improved once treatment with surgery was received.[24]

Although reconstructive surgery is considered the definitive treatment of a prolapse, not all women are candidates. Medical conditions may result in surgical risks that outweigh the benefits of repair. Some women are not interested in surgery and prefer a less invasive approach to treatment. Conservative treatment of POP includes expectant management consisting of weight loss, treatment of constipation, avoidance of heavy lifting, and pelvic floor muscle exercises (**Box 1**).[25] For some women, the use of a pessary is the best medical or personal option. It is important to assess the impact of prolapse on quality of life taking into consideration the age of the woman. For example, the impact of POP on quality of life for a younger woman may be different from that of an older woman.

PESSARY USE IN THE MANAGEMENT OF PELVIC ORGAN PROLAPSE

A pessary is a Food and Drug Administration-approved removable latex or silicone device manually inserted into the vagina by a provider or patient with the intent that the device supports the internal organs of the pelvis.

Table 3	
Epidemiology of pelvic organ prolapse	
Category	**Risk Factors**
Demographics	Age
	Genetics
Ethnicity	Hispanic (highest)
	Black (lowest)
Social status	Lower socioeconomic status
Disease/illness	Lung diseases
	Connective tissue disorders
Lifestyle/work related	Smoking (chronic cough)
	Jobs (repetitive heavy lifting)
	Obesity
	Impact to pelvic floor (exercise or sports)
Obstetric	Pregnancy
	Prolonged labor
	Forceps delivery
	Infant birth weight
	Parity

The word, pessary, originates from the Greek word, "pess'os," alluding to an oval stone used in a board game similar to checkers.[26] The gold standard for nonsurgical treatment of POP is the pessary.[27] Pessaries have been successfully used for thousands of years, with the pomegranate being the oldest known pessary.[28] Historically, other materials used for POP include balls of wax, wool, linen, cotton, sponge, brass, cork, and rubber.[29] Present-day pessaries are made primarily of silicone, although a few are still made of latex.[30]

The American College of Obstetricians and Gynecologists recommend a pessary be offered as first line therapy to all women with symptomatic POP.[31] Pessary use is a common approach but is not well known or discussed among women. Approximately 85% of gynecologists[32] and close to 98% of urogynecologists treat POP with pessaries.[33] A survey of registered and advanced practice nurses who are members of the American College of Nurse-Midwives, the American urogynecologic Society Allied Health Section, and the Society of Urologic Nurses and Associates report they use pessaries for treatment at a rate of 86.4%.[34] Provider factors for not considering a pessary as a valid treatment option include lack of interest,[33] perceived difficulty in insertion, and a concern related to correct positioning.[31]

Pessaries provide immediate relief of symptoms and are a low-risk, cost-effective treatment.[35] Currently, 2 categories of pessaries are used: support (ring, lever, and Gehrung) and space filling (cube, Gellhorn, donut, and Inflatoball [Bioteque America, Inc, San Jose, CA]).[36] Pessaries come in a variety of shapes and sizes. Some of the most commonly used pessaries are the ring, Gellhorn, cube, and donut (**Figs. 1–4**). Women often describe pessaries as life changing and miraculous when it comes to symptom relief.[37] Patient factors contributing to underutilization of pessaries include lack of knowledge, negative impressions, and aversion to pessaries.[38]

A pessary may prevent progression of prolapse; however, long-term data are scant.[7] Reasons to consider a trial of pessary use include symptomatic prolapse and a patient's desire for nonsurgical intervention. For some women, the desire to postpone/delay surgical intervention or to have additional children may play a key factor in treatment options.[28,36,39]

Potential contraindications for pessary use include gynecologic factors, such as vaginal or pelvic infection, endometriosis, vaginal atrophy, persistent vaginal erosion, and exposed vagina mesh.[39] Women with a latex sensitivity cannot use the Inflatoball. Sexually active women who are unable to remove/reinsert the pessary[36] and women who may not be willing or able to follow-up as needed are not good candidates.[37]

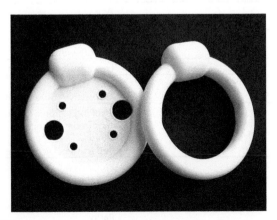

Fig. 1. Ring pessary.

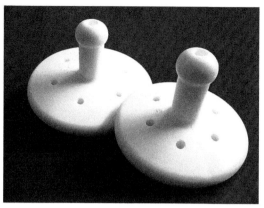

Fig. 2. Gellhorn pessary.

ATTITUDES AND PERCEPTIONS TOWARD PESSARY USE

Assessing patient and family knowledge of and experience with pessaries can reveal opinions, existing beliefs, and perceptions that create barriers to treatment. In a recent study of women presenting to a tertiary clinic, few had heard of pessaries, and those who had prior knowledge expressed negative views and aversion to pessary use.[38] Family and cultural attitudes may influence decisions for use. For example, among Thai women, the opinion of family members was an important factor for decision making and ultimate pessary acceptance.[40] Another consideration for pessary fitting and use relates to women reporting a history of sexual violence. Those women and women with a history of posttraumatic stress disorder and some veterans report more pain, distress, fear, discomfort, and embarrassment with pelvic examinations a potential strong deterrent to pessary use.[41–43]

FITTING AND ONGOING PESSARY USE

The goals of pessary fitting and ongoing treatment are symptom improvement, patient comfort, retention of the pessary during activities, and non-obstruction of urination and defecation during toileting.[44] There are no clear guidelines for fitting, follow-up

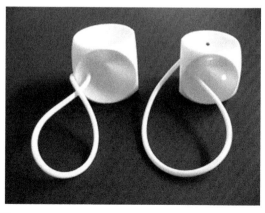

Fig. 3. Cube pessary.

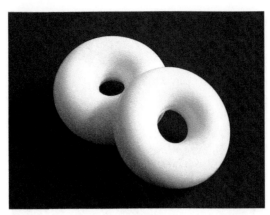

Fig. 4. Donut pessary.

or management of pessaries,[45] therefore many providers rely on expert opinion,[32,33] as well as personal experience. For example, approximately 70% of nurse providers who fit pessaries routinely scheduled return visits every 3 months, regardless of pessary type.[34] Manufacturers of pessaries propose follow-up of every 4 to weeks.[46] Overall, rates of success with pessary fittings and use in symptomatic women range from 41%[47] to 90%.[48]

There are no specific factors that might predict successful fitting and ongoing use of a pessary[49]; however, overall pessaries are well tolerated. Reports indicate, women who use low dose estrogen therapy, and have a prior history of surgery for prolapse repair via the abdominal approach, as opposed to vaginal surgery, are most successful in having a pessary fit properly and in tolerating ongoing use.[50] Patient satisfaction rates are higher in older women[49] with no prior pelvic surgery;[51] and in women with high parity who have less severe prolapse, and no urinary incontinence.[52] Unsuccessful fittings and inability to use a pessary occurs in a woman with a short vaginal length (<6 cm), wide vaginal introitus (>4 fingerbreadths), or previous hysterectomy. In addition, concurrent POP and urinary incontinence, younger age, and obesity can also predict fitting difficulty.[53]

SIDE EFFECTS AND COMPLICATIONS OF PESSARY USE

Common side effects of pessary use are vaginal discharge and odor. Common problems with pessary use are erosion of vaginal tissues due to poor vaginal estrogenization, incorrect type of pessary, poorly fitting pessary, and failure to present for follow-up care. Complications of pessary use include bacterial vaginitis, de novo stress incontinence, vaginal bleeding, ulceration of the vagina, and the pessary becoming imbedded in the cervix or migrating into the uterus. Severe complications are rare but preventable. These include fecal impaction, hydronephrosis with urosepsis, vesicovaginal and rectovaginal fistula, visceral obstruction, and cancer.[51]

ASSESSMENT AND DIAGNOSIS

Women who present for symptoms or signs of POP may also have other pelvic floor issues, such as incontinence of bowel and bladder, dyspareunia, incomplete bladder emptying, vaginal atrophy, infections, or vaginal cancers. Therefore, in addition to performing a comprehensive gynecologic history and focused physical examination, a comprehensive genitourinary examination is essential. The information obtained from the history and physical may uncover neurologic, endocrine, gastrointestinal, urogenital, or musculoskeletal disorders, which may require additional workup, testing, surgery, or referral.

MEDICAL AND SOCIAL HISTORY

When considering a pessary, an in-depth health history should focus on age, weight, symptoms, chronic illnesses, and medications as well as gynecologic and surgical components. An assessment of each symptom should be evaluated separately and should include onset, duration, severity, and alleviating and precip-itating factors as well as any prior treatments.[54] Chronic illnesses limiting range of motion, such as arthritis, fibromyalgia, and multiple sclerosis, should be taken into consideration before pessary treatment is considered, because limited range of motion and poor hand function may prevent self-management. Functional sta-tus—the ability to perform activities of daily life, such as bathing, dressing, toileting, transferring, and maintaining continence—should be appraised. Physical limita-tions, however, are not an absolute contraindication to pessary fitting and use. Women with the inability to care for a pessary may require more frequent follow-up visits.

Women with pessaries need regularly scheduled follow-up visits. This may be a pro-hibitive factor for women who are unable to transport themselves or who have cogni-tive impairment. Therefore, a family member or caregiver must have a firm understanding that a burden of care is associated with pessary use.

Literacy, language, and health literacy assessments can help assure comprehen-sion and adherence. Written instructions provide aid for women with poor recall or dif-ficulty following verbal instructions. When there is a concern related to memory loss, memory screening should be assessed using memory and thinking skills tools. Screening tools meeting the accepted criteria by the Alzheimer's Foundation of America that are quick, effective, and validated include the General Practitioner Assessment of Cognition, Mini-Cog, Memory Impairment Screen, and Brief Alz-heimer's Screen (nationalmemoryscreening.org).[55]

A social history may uncover past or current tobacco use, which may contribute to prolapse. An appraisal of occupational and recreational activities that may have contributed to the onset of prolapse, worsen pelvic floor symptoms, and make retain-ing a pessary difficult should be made. In addition, a review of living arrangements and availability of transportation is needed.

MEDICATIONS

A medication history and review of all current medications and herbal products are impor-tant and often overlooked when considering the use of a pessary. Although there are few if any studies examining the direct effects of medications, other than topical estrogen on the vaginal epithelium, some consideration should be given to the potential side effects of corticosteroids, anticoagulants, and herbal medications as these medications have been known to cause easy bleeding and bruising of the skin which may give rise to complications.

GYNECOLOGIC AND SURGICAL HISTORY

The gynecologic history informs the provider of pelvic cancers, labor, delivery, parity, and complications from childbirth as well as menopause and current sexual activity. Lack of hormone replacement and prior pessary use or prolapse treatment along with a surgical history may limit pessary choice. This may also make fitting more difficult and, in some cases, may exclude fitting and ongoing use altogether.

PHYSICAL EXAMINATION

A general examination is warranted. Adequate vision and depth perception are important for self-management and can prevent vaginal tissue injury and vaginal bleeding caused by inability to see a torn or damaged pessary. Lung conditions may cause chronic cough, a contributor to prolapse and a hindrance to pessary retainment. Flexibility to bend or squat, allowing the adequate knee and hip motion needed to insert and remove a pessary, should be assessed.

Assessing for prolapse can be performed in the lithotomy or in the standing position, but for an adequate pelvic examination, the woman must be able to abduct the thighs. This may be difficult for women with hip flexion contractures from injuries resulting in paraplegia or from neurologic conditions, such as cerebral palsy. External vaginal inspection may be all that is necessary to determine if a prolapse is present. A stenotic vagina may be readily seen on visual inspection and may prevent a speculum or digital examination.

Inspect for and document any discoloration, inflammation, irritation, discharge, rash, and lesions. A uniform system should be used to document the description and to communicate the type of prolapse, grade, and compartment. Maximum protrusion should be documented by the examiner to replicate that of the patient during daily activities.[21] In addition to assessment, it is important to remember that vaginal atrophy and bleeding or dry friable tissue may require treatment with vaginal moisturizers or topical vaginal estrogen before fitting can take place[56] (**Table 4**).

PSYCHOSOCIAL CONSIDERATIONS OF PESSARY USE

Due to the necessity for frequent follow-up care, financial concerns should be assessed, especially if the pessary care is to be managed by the provider. Copays may become a burden for women on fixed income. The cost of estrogen products to prevent pessary complications and promote patient comfort may also be prohibitive to some women. Transportation availability and cost may be factors if long distance travel is required or a pay for services is needed for follow up visits.

FOLLOW OF CARE CONSIDERATIONS

Follow-up varies by practice setting and is based on manufacturer recommendations, observational studies, surveys, and case studies. Therefore, expert opinion has become best practice.[46] Follow-up is tailored to the woman, based on patient and provider comfort levels, type of pessary inserted, and appearance of vaginal mucosa. Social support from family and the living situation should be assessed. Availability and willingness of the family to participate in care are essential. Contact information of the patient, caregiver, family member, and/or neighbor must be documented to prevent loss to follow-up.

COUNSELING PATIENTS AND CAREGIVERS ABOUT PESSARY CARE

Any woman with a pessary must be educated and informed of the signs and symptoms of pessary complications, in particular, increased discomfort, vaginal bleeding, and a change in normal voiding habits. Patient education related to pessary care and use varies among providers. In a study of pessary use for POP in the Netherlands,

Table 4
Evaluation of the pessary candidate

Component	Areas of Investigation

Bodily function	Vision
	  Visual acuity and depth perception
	Hearing
	  Fitting/maintenance instructions

Disease/illness	Lung diseases Connective tissue disorders Pelvic cancer/radiation Obesity
Lifestyle/work	Smoking (chronic cough) Jobs (repetitive heavy lifting) Impact to pelvic floor (exercise or sports)
Obstetric	Pregnancy Parity Prolonged labor Forceps delivery Cesarean section Infant birth weight Sexual activity
Medications	Corticosteroids Anticoagulants Herbals Estrogen products
Urinary symptoms	Sensation of incomplete bladder emptying Urinary hesitancy Urinary frequency Straining to void Spraying/split urinary stream
Vaginal symptoms	Vaginal pressure/pain/irritation/bleeding Abdominal pressure Sensation of vaginal bulge Prolapse interference with ambulation
Bowel assessment	Vaginal splinting to evacuate bowels Difficulty/straining with bowel movement Hard, bulky stools

Neurologic/motor	Mobility, balance, gait, range of motion
	Hand and finger dexterity/strength
	Sensation in the hands and pelvic floor
	Neurologic disease
	  Multiple sclerosis
	  Stroke
	  Arthritis

Psychosocial	Cognition Detection of dementia Living arrangements Caregiver/family support Compliant for maintenance Travel distance/transportation Financial/travel

all providers supplied information on the possibility of serious vaginal discharge and likelihood of vaginal blood loss,[56] but this may not be true elsewhere.

Providers who fit pessaries must consider the patient to be under active care as long as she uses the pessary. Documentation in the medical record of efforts to reach the woman, family or caregiver is important. Currently, there is no consensus for standardized regimens for follow-up. Practices vary according to self-management versus provider management, type of pessary, reason for use of a pessary, and condition of vaginal epithelium. Provider experience and comfort level with pessary fitting may also be factors in choosing recommended follow-up frequency. Strong consideration should be given for a method to identify women with a pessary when mental status and health decline. A medical identification band or bracelet, inclusion of the pessary on the medication list, a note to the primary care provider, signing a consent, and giving a copy to a family member or care provider can be helpful in preventing long-term complications due to lack of follow-up.

SUMMARY

Pelvic prolapse significantly affects quality of life, sexuality, and body image. Nurse providers who neglect to ask about symptoms of prolapse and who do not perform a pelvic examination during the overall assessment and care of a woman may be missing the opportunity to detect prolapse. Components of a visit should include a history, pelvic examination, pessary fitting (if indicated), and patient education. Thus, women who have POP present special challenges because patient visits can be lengthy and time consuming. Lengthy visits may be discouraged in a practice where a productivity model is in place.

In addition, caregiver and family involvement in decision making, maintenance, and support is necessary for safe, effective pessary care and follow-up. Moving forward it will be important to create a universally accepted method to describe prolapse and to develop standardize findings to enhance ongoing care.

REFERENCES

1. Haylen BT, Maher CF, Barber MD, et al. An International Urogynecological Association (IUGA)/International Continence Society (ICS) report on the terminology for female pelvic organ prolapse (POP). Neurourol Urodyn 2016;35:137–68.
2. Cordozo L, Staskin D. Textbook of female urology and urogynecology. 4th edition. Boca Raton (FL): Taylor & Francis Group, LLC; 2017.
3. Rosenblum N, Eilber KS, Rodriguez LV, et al. Anatomy of pelvic support. In: Appell RA, Sand PK, Raz S, editors. Female urology, urogynecology, and voiding dysfunction. Boca Raton (FL): Taylor and Francis; 2005.
4. Bump MD, Neubauer NL, Klein-Olarte V. Can we screen for pelvic organ prolapse and pelvic floor dysfunction. Am J Obstet Gynecol 1996;175(1):10–7.
5. Beckly I, Harris N. Pelvic organ prolapse: a urology perspective. J Clin Urol 2013; 6(2):68–76.
6. Nygaard IE, Shaw JM, Bardsley T, et al. Lifetime physical activity and pelvic organ prolapse in middle-aged women. Am J Obstet Gynecol 2014;210(5): 477.e1-12.
7. Tezelli-Borlolini MA. Genetics of pelvic organ prolapse: crossing the bridge between bench and bedside in urogynecologic research. Int Urogynecol J 2011; 22:1211–99.
8. Hendrix SL, Clark A, Nygaard I, et al. Pelvic organ prolapse in the Women's Health Initiative: gravity and gravidity. Am J Obstet Gynecol 2002;186(6):1160–6.

9. Handa VL, Lockhart ME, Fielding JR, et al. Racial difference in pelvic anatomy by magnetic resonance imaging. Obstet Gynecol 2008;111:914–20.

10. Kudish BI, Iglesia CB, Gutman RE, et al. Risk factors for prolapse development in white, black, and Hispanic women. Female Pelvic Med Reconstr Surg 2012; 17(2):80–90.

11. Sze EH, Sherard GB, Dolezal JM. Pregnancy, labor, delivery, and pelvic organ prolapse. Obstet Gynecol 2002;100(5):981–6.

12. Allen-Brady K, Cannon-Albright LA, Farnham JM, et al. Evidence for pelvic organ prolapse predisposition genes on chromosomes 10 and 17. Am J Obstet Gynecol 2015;212(6):771.e1-7.

13. Bump RC, Norton PA. Epidemiology and natural history of pelvic floor dysfunction. Obstet Gynecol Clin North Am 1998;25(4):723–46.

14. Giri A, Hartmann KE, Helbruge JN, et al. Obesity and pelvic organ prolapse: a systematic review and meta-analysis of observational studies. Am J Obstet Gynecol 2017;217(1):11–26.e3.

15. MacLennan AH, Taylor AW, Wilson DH, et al. The prevalence of pelvic floor disorders and their relationship to gender, age, parity and mode of delivery. BJOG 2000;107(12):1460–70.

16. Lukacz ES, Lawrence JM, Contreras R, et al. Parity, mode of delivery, and pelvic floor disorders. Obstet Gynecol 2006;107(6):1253–60.

17. Zhu L, Bian XM, Long Y, et al. Role of different childbirth strategies on pelvic organ prolapse and stress urinary incontinence: a prospective study. Chin Med J (Engl) 2008;121(3):213–5.

18. Lindo FM, Carr ES, Reyes M, et al. Randomized trial of cesarean vs vaginal delivery for effects on the pelvic floor in squirrel monkeys. Am J Obstet Gynecol 2015;213(5):735.e1-8.

19. Carley ME, Schaffer J. Urinary incontinence and pelvic organ prolapse in women with Marfan or Ehlers-Danlos syndrome. Am J Obstet Gynecol 2000;182(5):1021.

20. McIntosh LJ, Mallett VT, Frahm JD, et al. Gynecologic disorders in women with Ehlers-Danlos syndrome. J Soc Gynecol Investig 1995;2(3):165e1-6.

21. Barber MD, Lambers AR, Visco AG, et al. Effect of patient position on clinical evaluation of pelvic organ prolapse. Obstet Gynecol 2000;96(1):18–22.

22. Thakar R, Stanton S. Management of genital prolapse. BMJ 2002;324(7348): 1258–62.

23. Lowder JJ, Ghetti C, Nekolajski C, et al. Body image perceptions in women with pelvic organ prolapse: a qualitative study. Am J Obstet Gynecol 2011;204(441): 1–5.

24. Ghetti C, Lowder JL, Ellison R, et al. Depressive symptoms in women seeking surgery for pelvic organ prolapse. Int Urogynecol J 2010;21(7):855–60.

25. Guidelines for the Use of Support Pessaries in the Management of Pelvic Organ Prolapse. International Centre for Allied Health Evidence, 2012. Available at: https://www.clinicalguidelines.gov.au. Accessed September 21, 2017.

26. Oliver R, Thakar R, Sultan AH. The history and usage of the vaginal pessary: a review. Eur J Obstet Gynecol Reprod Biol 2011;156:125–30.

27. Alas AN, Bresee C, Eilber K, et al. Measuring the quality of care provided to women with pelvic organ prolapse. Am J Obstet Gynecol 2015;212(4):471.e1-9.

28. Miller DS. Chapter 39. Contemporary use of the pessary. Gynecology and Obstetrics. Volume 1. Philadelphia: Lippincott Williams & Wilkins; 2004. p. 1–16.

29. Shah SM, Sultan AH, Thakar R. The history and evolution of pessaries for pelvic organ prolapse. Int Urogynecol J 2006;17:170–5.

30. Bash KL. Review of vaginal pessaries. Obstet Gynecol Surv 2000;55(7):455–60.

31. ACOG Committee on Practice Bulletins–Gynecology. ACOG Practice bulletin no. 85: pelvic organ prolapse. Obstet Gynecol 2007;110:717–29.
32. Pott-Grinstein E, Newcomer JR. Gynecologist' patterns of prescribing pessaries. J Reprod Med 2001;46:205–8.
33. Cundiff GW, Weidner AC, Visco AG, et al. A survey of pessary use by members of the American Urogynecologic Society. Obstet Gynecol 2000;95:931–5.
34. O'Dell K, Atnip S, Hooper GL, et al. Pessary care practices of nurse-providers in the United States. Female Pelvic Med Reconstr Surg 2016;22(4):261–6.
35. Atnip SD. Pessary use and management for pelvic organ prolapse. Obstet Gynecol Clin North Am 2009;36(3):541–53.
36. Trowbridge ER, Fenner DE. Practicalities and pitfalls of pessaries in older women. Clin Obstet Gynecol 2007;50(3):709–19.
37. Storey S, Ashton M, Price S, et al. Women's experiences with vaginal pessary use. J Adv Nurs 2009;65(11):2350–7.
38. Brown LK, Fenner DE, Delancey JOL, et al. Defining patient knowledge and perceptions of vaginal pessaries for prolapse and incontinence. Female Pelvic Med Reconstr Surg 2016;22(2):93–7.
39. Clemons JL, Aguilar VC, Sokol ER, et al. Patient characteristics that are associated with continued pessary use versus surgery after 1 year. Am J Obstet Gynecol 2004;191(1):159–64.
40. Mungpooklang T, Bunyavejchevin S. Attitudes towards use among Thai women with pelvic organ prolapse. J Obstet Gynaecol Res 2017;1–5. https://doi.org/10.1111/jog.13374.
41. Robohm JS, Buttenheim M. The gynecological care experience of adult survivors of childhood sexual abuse: a preliminary investigation. Women Health 1997;24(3):59–75.
42. Lang AJ, Rodgers CS, Laffaye C, et al. Sexual trauma, posttraumatic stress disorder, and health behavior. Behav Med 2003;28(4):150–8.
43. Weitlauf JC, Frayne SM, Finney JW, et al. Sexual violence, posttraumatic stress disorder, and the pelvic examination: how do beliefs about the safety, necessity, and utility of the examination influence patient experiences? J Womens Health 2010;19(7):1271–80.
44. Atnip S, O'Dell K. Vaginal support pessaries: Indications for use and fitting strategies. Urol Nurs 2012;32(3):114–24.
45. Alpern M, Khan A, Dubina E, et al. Patterns of pessary care and outcomes for medicare beneficiaries with pelvic organ prolapse. Female Pelvic Med Reconstr Surg 2013;19(3):142–7.
46. Bioteque America Incorporated. Ver. 2.303. 2011. Available at: www.bioteque.com. Accessed September 26, 2017.
47. Mutone MF, Terry C, Hale DS, et al. Factors which influence the short-term success of pessary management of pelvic organ prolapse. Am J Obstet Gynecol 2005;193:89–94.
48. Cundiff GW, Amundsen CL, Bent AE, et al. The PESSRI Study: symptom relief outcomes of a randomized crossover trial of the ring and Gellhourn pessaries. Am J Obstet Gynecol 2007;196:405.e1-8.
49. Maito JM, Quam ZA, Craig E, et al. Predictors of successful pessary fitting and continued use in a nurse-midwifery pessary clinic. J Midwifery Womens Health 2006;51:78–84.
50. Hanson LAM, Schultz JA, Flood CG, et al. Vaginal pessaries in managing women with pelvic organ prolapse and urinary incontinence: patient characteristics and

factors contributing to success. Int Urogynecol J Pelvic Floor Dysfunct 2006; 17(2):155–9.

51. Nguyen JN, Jones CR, Krissovich M. Pessary treatment of pelvic relaxation: factors affecting successful fitting and continued use. J Wound Ostomy Continence Nurs 2005;32(4):255–63.

52. Wu V, Farrell SA, Baskett TF, et al. A simplified protocol for pessary management. Obstet Gynecol 1997;90(6):990–4.

53. Clemons JL, Aguilar VC, Tillinghast TA, et al. Risk factors associated with an unsuccessful pessary fitting trial in women with pelvic organ prolapse. Am J Obstet Gynecol 2004;190(2):345–50.

54. Marchese K. Improving evidence-based practice: use of the POP-Q system for the assessment of pelvic organ prolapse. Urol Nurs 2009;29(40):216–23.

55. Alzheimers Foundation of America. Available at: http://alzfdn.org/memory-screening. Accessed September 26, 2017.

56. Velzel J, Roovers JP, Van der Vaart CH, et al. A nationwide survey concerning practices in pessary use for pelvic organ prolapse in The Netherlands: identifying needs for further research. Int Urogynecol J 2015;26:1453–8.

Moving?

Make sure your subscription moves with you!

To notify us of your new address, find your **Clinics Account Number** (located on your mailing label above your name), and contact customer service at:

Email: journalscustomerservice-usa@elsevier.com

800-654-2452 (subscribers in the U.S. & Canada)
314-447-8871 (subscribers outside of the U.S. & Canada)

Fax number: 314-447-8029

Elsevier Health Sciences Division
Subscription Customer Service
3251 Riverport Lane
Maryland Heights, MO 63043

*To ensure uninterrupted delivery of your subscription, please notify us at least 4 weeks in advance of move.

Printed and bound by CPI Group (UK) Ltd, Croydon, CR0 4YY

03/10/2024

01040394-0016